# “R

## and the

# Work Related Upper Limb Disorders

Dr P. V. A. MACLOUGHLIN

MRCS, LRCP, DIH, PhD

PETERBOROUGH PRESS

First published in 1998 by
The Peterborough Press
56 North Twelth Street
Central Milton Keynes,
MK9 3BT



ISBN 0-9535070-0-9

A

**Chelsea** *Production*

Printed and bound in Great Britain by
Aztech Creative Print
32–33 Minton Park, Potters Lane
Kiln Farm, Milton Keynes
MK11 3HG

CONTENTS

# ILLUSTRATIONS

*Between pages 34 – 35*



Illustrations based on *Grays Anatomy,* 30th Edition (1949).

## ACKNOWLEDGEMENTS

I should like to thank the following people who have supported and encouraged the writing of this book.

Wendi Brownlie, my secretary, for all the hours spent in typing and retyping the manuscript and coordinating everyone involved with the publishing of the book.

Marika Johnson whose enormous contributions to the RSI Support Group should be given much more recognition and who has given me enormous help and encouragement throughout this project.

Wendy Lawrence who, as a representative of the RSI Association, encouraged and supported this project from the very beginning and also made some very constructive criticisms of the early drafts of the book.

Nicola McGregor who read the manuscript at the proof stage and made many helpful suggestions.

Mr Jeffrey Palmer of Cromptons, solicitors, who gave up his valuable time to proof read the manuscript and advise on various legal aspects of the book.

Julian Wesolowski for producing the layout and typesetting and for always being on hand to advise on matters relating to the production of the book.

Barry and Terry and all the staff at Aztech Creative Print for their help and advice on all the printing aspects of the book.

# FOREWORD

The syndromes now known in the UK as work related upper limb disorders (WRULDs) are recognised by many other names both within the UK and abroad. Repetitive strain injury (RSI); cumulative trauma disorder (CTD) in the USA; repetitive motion injury (RMI) in Canada; occupational cervicobrachial disorder (OCD) in Sweden and Japan; and occupational overuse disorder (OOD) in Australia. There are others. In reality these terms cover a wide spectrum of physical and physiological responses in the soft tissues of the hands, wrists, arms, shoulders and neck often associated with abnormalities of posture and, later, by a psychological overlay. Such physical and psychological responses can also manifest themselves differently in individuals, even though the occupational factors are the same.

None of the above names are entirely satisfactory but in the absence of anything better WRULD must suffice to describe what are essentially overuse or misuse syndromes which for centuries have been recognised under many different names – names often associated with local crafts and industries – and brought on by the heavy physical burdens laid upon the skeleton and soft tissues by the demands of agriculture and heavy manual labour. The change from an agricultural to a largely industrialised and manufacturing based society changing, in turn, towards a service based economy has currently led to a much greater emphasis on computer and word processor skills and to the simple, but constantly repeated movements which these skills entail. Likewise in industry much of the work previously carried out by skilled workers has been taken over by technology with many of those manufacturing and industrial processes which continue to need a human input being of a simpler repetitive nature, often carried out thousands of times an hour and sometimes in an unsuitable working environment.

The human skeleton and soft tissues were not designed to meet these constantly repeated movements, forced or otherwise, which – if persevered with – can provoke physiological reactions in the upper limbs characterised by numbness, tingling, swelling, weakness, discomfort or pain: the syndrome now known as WRULD. Some conditions which are involved in this syndrome are medically well defined and understood; others are not.

This book will attempt to describe the clinical manifestations of the various forms of WRULD found in the Western world; to show how they arise; their investigation, diagnosis, treatment and prevention; and give a brief outline of the current medico-legal situation and workers' compensation litigation.

This work is not a comprehensive medical text book and is aimed at non-specialist medical practitioners, health workers and lawyers working in the medico-legal field. It is hoped however, by the avoidance of unnecessary medical jargon, and the provision of a comprehensive glossary, that a wider audience – particularly the WRULD sufferers themselves – will be helped to understand a group of increasingly common complaints.

*Chapter 1*

# Historical Perspective

It is conventional to take Bernardino Ramazzini (1633–1714) as the first physician to take an interest in the diseases of workers and to describe – in *de Morbis Artificum Diatriba* – the occupationally related upper limb disorders.

Certainly there is no question that Ramazzini was the father of occupational medicine – even though work related upper limb disorders have been with us since man first became a tool-maker. It is probably not too fanciful to imagine stone age flint knappers complaining of aches and pains in their hands and forearms after long working sessions of tap, tap, tapping one flint against another. Little has changed over the years and work related upper limb disorders, as seen by today's occupational health physicians, rheumatologists or orthopaedic surgeons, are still, essentially, soft tissue injuries reflecting the varying occupational demands made, most commonly, on the bones, muscles, tendons, blood vessels and nerves of the hands, arms, neck and shoulders. Work related upper limb disorders, and other occupationally related conditions, have been recognised over the centuries to faithfully reflect the type and changing nature of industry, commerce and trade. Each occupation had, and still has, techniques and manual skills peculiar to its own and, inevitably, many of these working activities have had specifically adverse effects on the human frame.

Donald Hunter, the doyen of British occupational medicine, in his monumental *Diseases of Occupations*, lists hundreds of adverse reactions to occupational and industrial working conditions, and it was Hunter who, following on Ramazzini 300 years before, taught generations of medical students to ask their patients the simple but often very revealing question 'what is your occupation?'

Hunter showed that those whose work involved pressure, friction or repeated slight blows developed occupational bursae (sacks of fluid) known locally under such names as weaver's bottom, miner's elbow, housemaid's knee and humper's lump, all of which describe the development of bursae filled with synovial fluid as a protection to the underlying bony prominence. With the passing of the working practices which produced them, many of these conditions became of historical interest only whilst, at the same time, other conditions appeared reflecting the development of new working activities.

Often associated with the occupational bursae were traumatic changes in the tendons, or their coverings, called tenosynovitis. This condition can be due to the adverse effects of constantly repeated small movements which, whilst individually of little importance, have a cumulatively pathological effect. These fine movements, particularly those involving grasping actions, or nipping between thumb and fingers accompanied by quick pronation/supination movements of the forearm, were a frequent cause of pain in the hands and forearms.

Carpenters, upholsterers, linoleum fitters, and others who hammer nails all day were effected; also tea, tobacco and food packers and others who repeatedly opened and closed the lids of boxes; sewing machine operators, workers on the assembly line in the motor car industry – especially when a spanner or a hand held tool is used in a repetitive manner – agricultural workers – especially those who used a sickle or scythe, cane cutters, makers of fishing nets, all were liable to develop traumatic tenosynovitis.

It is probable that all industrial and manufacturing activities of the past which involved any form of repetitive movement – and most did – had their own locally known overuse syndromes which were known by such names as 'craft palsies', 'occupational palsies', 'occupational spasms' and 'occupational cramps'.

Hunter describes how the hands and arms were affected in writers, telegraphists, cotton twisters, tailors, drapers, seamstresses, sail makers, knitters, hairdressers, ironers, bowlers, metal workers, hammer men, turners, engravers, gold beaters, cabinet makers, lock smiths, tin smiths, nail makers, masons, painters, enamellers, compositors, watchmakers, shoemakers, saddlers, sailors, fencers, diamond cutters, money counters, letter sorters, cigarette rollers, cigar makers, pianists, organists, violinists, cellists, harpists, comptometer workers, waiters, florists, artificial flower makers, folders of newspapers, milkers of cows – and many others.

Most of these occupations involved rapid repetitive movements of short range using one or both hands. The movements concerned are complex, perfected by education and practice, necessitate a high degree of precision and co-ordination, and may involve as many as 600 repetitions of movements a minute. Hunter noticed that the soft tissue disorder was likely to manifest itself when the worker returned from holiday or was called upon, either willingly or otherwise, to exceed a certain level of performance – situations which still prevail today even though the nature of the working processes may have changed.

In 1920 Bridge described a form of occupational cramp in the Lancashire cotton trade which could suddenly attack cotton twisters of many years' experience. In joining the threads of a warp – the weaving of which had been completed – to the threads of a new warp the two ends are twisted between the flexed left thumb and the dorsum of the left index finger. An experienced man could join 2,000 ends in one hour, each warp having between 2,000 and 2,500 threads. The symptoms were pain, cramp and loss of power in the affected muscles, with about 50% of patients showing wasting of the left thenar eminence. It was a disability causing much loss of earning power in the men affected, and anxiety made it worse. Treatment by massage, exercises and rest although alleviating the condition, did not cure it. In severe cases an entire change of employment was found to be necessary. This type of work is no longer with us but other forms of work involving similar constantly repeated hand movements have taken its place.

Word processor operators may carry out as many as 25,000 fine keyboard movements an hour under employer pressure or in order to achieve a bonus level – with work related upper limb disorders likely to develop when key depressions exceed 10,000 an hour.

Mail sorters may perform more than 64,000 key strokes per day; turkey carcase processors may perform more than 12,000 cuts per shift; tobacco workers can carry out up to 2,000 manipulations per hour and workers in the pottery industry can deal with 1,500 to 2,000 hand held items an hour.

Nevertheless, in the 1990s it is the keyboard operator who comes forward as the most vulnerable occupational group and seems likely to be even more at risk in the next century as computers became an increasingly accepted part of daily life, both occupationally and domestic.

But in previous centuries it was writer's cramp which was the main problem and it is surprising how the description of writer's cramp by Ramazzini (1713), Sir Charles Bell (1830), Dr G. V. Poore (1877), Dr W. R. Gowers (1893) and Sir William Osler (1900) described the hand pains suffered by telegraphic workers; and *Telegraphist's Cramp* (HMSO 1919) – as well as a great many other nineteenth century papers on writer's cramp under its various names in the USA, Germany,

France and Italy – have so many things in common with the 1998 complaints of computer keyboard operators.

In his descriptions of the *Disease of Scribes and Notaries* Ramazzini states that:

> 'That there was a far greater number of scribes and notaries among ancients than there is in our day because of the invention of the art of printing, is certain: nevertheless, everyone knows that in every city and town there are many persons who support themselves and their families solely by writing. Incessant driving of the pen over paper causes intense fatigue of the hand and the whole arm because of the continuous and almost tonic strain on the muscles and tendons which in the course of time result in failure of power in the right hand. An acquaintance of mine, a notary by profession, still living, used to spend his whole life continually engaged in writing, and he made a good deal of money by it. First he began to complain of intense fatigue in the whole arm, but no remedy could relieve this, and finally the whole right arm became completely paralysed. In order to offset this infirmity he began to train himself to write with the left hand, but it was not very long before it too was attacked by the same malady. But what tortures these workers suffered most acutely is the intense and incessant application of the mind, for in such work as this the whole brain, its nerves and fibres must be kept constantly on the stretch; hence ensues loss of tonus. From this result headaches, heavy colds, sore throats and fluxes to the eyes from keeping them fixed on the paper: those who suffer most from these ailments are book keepers and accountants, as they are called, for example those who hire themselves to work for

> merchants. Also we must reckon in the same category the private secretaries of princes. For weakness of the arm and the right hand it will be beneficial to apply rubbing but it should be rather gentle and done with oil of sweet almond to which you can add a small portion of brandy to strengthen the part affected. In winter they must take care not to let the hands grow numb from excessive cold, so they must be protected by good thick gloves.'

Much of what Ramazzini writes about writer's cramp can be equally applied to many of today's workers in industry and commerce and his drawing attention to the reduced number of scribes and notaries – with the invention of printing – has many parallels today as old technology gives way to new.

Writer's cramp however, remained a problem and Sir Charles Bell in 1830 was able to write an erudite description of the condition – which was also called 'Writing Neurosis', 'Scriveners Palsy' and 'Graphospasm'. Showing that systemic disease or local injury could precipitate symptoms.

Dr G. V. Poore physician to University College Hospital, London, also wrote a description of writer's cramp in 1877 drawing attention to pain, numbness, tingling, heaviness and fatigue of the arm which many of today's WRULD sufferers would recognise as their own symptoms. At the same time Dr Poore could find no signs of sensory loss or muscle wasting to support the symptoms – a limitation which persists today when the law states that:

> 'Unless the Plaintiff can show a condition with known pathology the mere fact that he or she suffers pain as a result of performing an activity in the course of employment does not permit recovery: actual injury must be shown as recognised by a body of medical opinion.'

In 1893 Dr W. R. Gowers also gave a classical description of the condition which he saw to be very much dependent on the way in which the pen was held and the muscles involved with its movements.

> 'The chief agent in the production of the malady is the act of writing, which has usually been excessive in degree. Hence the affection occurs chiefly among those who earn their living by writing, and clerks furnish the majority of cases. But it now and then occurs in persons who have not done an excessive amount of writing; and in such cases a powerful predisposing cause, such as anxiety or neuralgia, may commonly be traced. The occurrence of the disease is influenced less by the amount than by the manner of writing. There are in writing two chief elements: the way in which the pen is held, and the way in which the movements are effected. The mode in which the pen is held is comparatively unimportant; it is mode in which the pen is moved that chiefly determines the occurrence of the disease.
>
> 'Occasionally the onset is acute. Other delicate movements are not affected until late in the disorder, and it is striking how, asked to unlace his shoe with the affected hand, the patient performs this act to perfection. Power in the hand may be slightly impaired; wasting is exceptional. Sensory symptoms are usually prominent and rarely absent. A sense of fatigue in the hand is followed by spasm and dull pain, occasionally with local tenderness. The pain may be referred along the course of the nerves; paraesthesia may affect the fingers. The symptoms continue with the attempts to write. The sensory symptoms spread more than the motor. In about 50% of those who have learnt to write with the other

> hand, symptoms appear for a second time and may progress more rapidly in the second arm than in the first.
>
> 'No anatomical changes are known. Clearly the condition is one of central and not of local origin, since local weakness is only found to a degree comparable with spasm.
>
> 'The limitation of symptoms to the act of writing is diagnostic. Distinction must most often be made from painful and paralytic affections of the hand, including gradual hemiplegia, disseminated sclerosis, cervical tabes, radial palsy and even torsion-dystinia at its onset. Simple pain from excessive writing must also be distinguished. The prognosis is poor when the disorder is more established, if there are no extraneous causes other than writing and if complete rest from writing is impossible.
>
> 'Treatment, to be effective, must be early. Rest may relieve the symptoms within a month, but in well established cases six months will be required. Facility in writing with the unaffected hand is not difficult to acquire. A typewriter may be recommended for recalcitrant cases. Where there is pain, sedatives internally and locally are certainly of service. Electricity is of little use, but massage and exercises often relieve the spasm and pain.'

Here again the onset of this condition as described by Gower has many parallels in modern industry and commerce and his suggestions of avoidance and treatment reflect today's advice given by many medical practitioners as well as the TUC and the Unions.

The use of the Morse key soon led to a new type of occupational disability called 'telegraphists' cramp', and this became well known by the year 1880. The Morse key is a clumsy brass instrument, the knob of which is depressed by hand in areas of rapid movements which makes and breaks the circuit in such a way as to transmit the dots and dashes of the Morse code. In the 1919 *Report of the Departmental Committee on Telegraphists' Cramp* (HMSO) various objective factors – such as types of keys, length of service, hours of work and bad style – were reviewed. Even the physiological signs of cramp were shown to be indeterminate, as there might, or might not, be a visible spasm, and the disability in its objective manifestations could be specific to one letter, or selective for certain muscular activities, or associated with general muscular weakness. Morse key operators sometimes suddenly, sometimes gradually, become unable to control the movements required for using the Morse key. This would suggest some muscular difficulty due to the cumulative effect of the work, or to an initial weakness or to the introduction of some new factor. The muscular difficulty alone, however, is not disabling, as many telegraphists could carry on in spite of it.

On reading the HMSO report it is noticeable that scattered throughout – in connection with each suggested cause – are references to 'psychoneurosis', 'cramp subjects', 'neurasthenia', 'nervous instability', 'personal factors', 'temperamental factors', 'highly strung disposition', 'nervous temperament', and various other nervous or psychological conditions. Clearly the symptomotology could manifest itself in many different ways.

These psychological opinions about causation differ little from the opinions offered today about many workers – often women – who develop WRULDs and then are told their disability is due to 'constitutional' or 'emotional' factors. Many women do eventually demonstrate emotional or psychological problems but this is secondary to, not the cause of, the disability and reflect the considerable disruptions which WRULDs can, did in the past, and still do, bring to a sufferer's life.

Patients with telegraphists' cramp did not all show the same symptoms and two types of disability were described.

> 'There are those suffering from the general disability to use the arm after many years of sending; not only is the use of the telegraphic key or a pencil interfered with, but also most other actions which demand the use of the arm. The holding of a cup, or of a needle for sewing or knitting, is difficult or impossible; a glass if taken up may be dropped; even the handle of spade cannot be grasped. This disability may or may not be accompanied by pain, which may be localized in the wrist or may be general.' (*A description which will sound remarkably familiar to those keyboard operators in the 1990s who develop the non-specific pain syndrome.*)
>
> 'There are those who can neither send nor write but who can use the arm for other occupations. This group comprises very many individual variants – from ability to use the arm for anything except telegraphic work, through various grades of inability, to total disability.
>
> 'The sufferer feels innocent and may react with antagonism to those around him, or recognise his inefficiency but still feel powerless to alter it. Even if this state were the invariable sequence, a remedy would be relatively simple – namely, to accept such initial difficulties and take the telegraphist off. There are, however, many subjects who have admitted that they have had occasional difficulty with certain words and sequences, but that it has passed away; the mechanism of this passing away is obscure, but it probably involves improvement in general health, absence of the fear of cramp and temperamental stability. The fear of cramp is very real to many telegraphists and probably plays no small part in

> determining the attack, which, without this, might be temporary muscular tiredness, relieved by rest.'

Much of this is also only too familiar to those who deal with WRULDs in the 1990s reflecting as it does the physiological effect of the excessive demands made upon the soft tissues.

Mild cases of telegraphists's cramp recovered when prolonged rest was ordered, in many of the severe cases nothing short of an entire change of employment would cure the condition. The disappearance of anxiety obviously had a good influence on the prognosis. The problem was largely solved by mechanisation in the form of the tape machine. Automatic recording systems which are essentially letter-printing instruments came into extensive use in about 1880. The teleprinter was an electrically operated typewriter with a standard keyboard which replaced the Morse key almost universally. The extended use of the telephone also helped the situation.

In 1908 telegraphist's cramp was added to the schedule of diseases covered by the 1906 Workman's Compensation Act.

Much of the advice given to professional writers and telegraphist's in the nineteenth century in an attempt to help their painful hands is remarkably similar to the advice currently (1998) given by the Health and Safety Executive, and Trade Unions medical advisors to those suffering from work related upper limb disorders.

Just as scribes were replaced by printers, so typewriters reduced the need for handwritten records and were, in turn, forced to give way to computers and word processors. As there is thus a constant change in the nature of industrial and commercial processes so there are changes in the demands made upon the human body – and in the ill effects which those demands create.

Reliable epidemiological studies however, are difficult to obtain and the incidence of WRULDs in the general population is either unknown or anecdotal.

A Japanese study published in 1976[1] reported on the difference in the incidence of shoulder, arm and wrist and hand symptoms between office machine operators, cash register operators and other office workers. The findings suggested that the symptoms was directly related to muscle groups used, and postures adopted in the respective occupations. The authors also commented on evidence of increased general symptoms such as headache, fatigue and insomnia in the cash register operators as opposed to other groups. This was said to reflect psychological stress at work.

Other comparative studies in Switzerland,[2] Japan,[3] and Finland[4] have also demonstrated increased disorders of the upper limb in certain occupations that demand rapid, repetitive movements.

In Japan, an epidemic of occupational cervico-brachial disorders was reported between 1958 and 1982.[1,5,6,7,8,9] Workers affected included punch card perforators, typists, telephone operators, keyboard operators and process workers.[10] As a result of this high incidence of WRULDs (10% to 28% of workers affected, depending on the occupational group studied), the Japanese Ministry of Labour in 1964 introduced measures designed to counter the problem. Work guidelines or keyboard operators were laid down, allowing no more than 5 hours' work a day, a 10 minute rest break each hour and no more than 40,000 keystrokes a day (many operators without such guidelines may make more than 100,000 keystrokes a day). The introduction of these measures, along with job rotation, led to a reduction in the incidence of upper limb, notably arm and hand, repetition strain injuries.[1]

Other countries have also reported on the incidence of RSI in different occupational groups. Much literature has emerged from Australia where RSI reached epidemic proportions in the 1980s with wide media and television coverage. The number of successful occupational claims for WRULDs in New South Wales increased from 762 in 1978–1979 to 2,263 in

1981–1982.[10] The incidence of WRULDs was far greater than these figures suggest, and the resulting disability and subsequent claims for compensation led to a rapid increase in the insurance premiums. This often exceeded 5% and occasionally was 30% of the payroll costs which, as in the USA, had a dramatic effect on the ability of some companies to compete in world markets.[11]

In 1985, the RSI Committee of the Australian National Occupational Health and Safety Commission reported that the largest number of cases of RSI occurred in the occupational groups tradesmen, production process workers and labourers, followed by clerical workers, service, sports and recreational workers, sales workers, farmers, fishermen, and workers in the timber industry.[12] Other published reports demonstrated the high incidence of symptomatic RSI in the general working population – up to 78% of workers studies in one paper.[13,14]

In the USA by 1991 Cumulative Trauma Disorder – WRULDs in the UK – accounted for 18% of all recorded occupational illnesses. By 1989 this had increased to 52% of recorded occupational illness – and resulted in medical costs of more than $22 billion[15] – and in the 1990s CTD have continued to account for more than 50% of all occupational disease or illness reported in the USA.[16] There are estimates which suggest that 50% of the entire American workforce could be affected by CTDs by the year 2000.[18]

WRULDs are thus taken very seriously in the USA. The Clinton administration has proposed extensive health and safety regulations to control WRULDs that cost an estimated $100 billion (£62.5 billion) a year in lost work time.[19]

The USA Labour Department's Occupational Safety and Health Administration has completed a draft standard on the work environment and its affect on efficiency which will cover more than 120 million workers in all but the smallest companies.[20]

When implemented, employers will have to examine every job with an eye to potential upper limb problem. Once identified, the employer will have 60 days to put it right. This might involve simple changes to the schedule of a typist suffering wrist strain, or the redesign of assembly line equipment. The American National Association of Manufacturers has formed a lobby to assure that the new standard is to its liking. So far 185 have joined its 'Coalition on Ergonomics'.

In the two years preceding the writing of this book the author has dealt with work related conditions of the upper limbs from a wide spectrum of workers including computer operators, users of printing machines, counters of bank notes, users of staple guns, computer mouse users, upholsterers, onion sorters and baggers, chicken carcase processors, farmers, stackers of bank note paper, tyre fitters, hairdressers, journalists, musicians, blanket folders, many different types of workers in the pottery industry, lockers of doors, supermarket check out operators, laundry workers, potato sorters, vibration machine operators, labourers, many different types of assembly line workers and has, probably for the first time, recorded a new local craft name 'Doffer's elbow' – which is a type of epicondylitis specific to men (see case histories).

Although there are still many thousands of different industrial processes involving manual handling, and there have been many different names given to the ill effects these processes have on the human frame, there are a finite number of muscles and associated anatomical structures which can be involved.

Diagnosis and litigation is still however, bedevilled by the difficulty in demonstrating measurable pathological changes and more research, and probably into nerve dysfunction, must be carried out before acceptable parameters of diagnosis can be established.

With knowledge however, of the relevant anatomy – and the skill to analyse the nature of the hand and arm movements

– those muscles groups involved and their neurological components can be identified and related to the unacceptable working practices which damage them and their associated structures.

In summary, the relationship between working procedures and upper limb disorders is not a new phenomena. It has been with us, in one form of another, since man first became the tool maker, always reflecting the ever changing nature of work, in agricultural, industry, technology and commerce.

In recent years sensational media coverage, ill informed comment, the availability of state benefits and worker's compensation have all influenced the epidemiology of upper limb disorders but these factors are not the cause of the disorders they are merely part of the effect.

The vast world wide literature on WRULDs can, and is, used to prove almost any point of view for, or against, the relationship between work and upper limb disorders and the supporters of the existence of WRULDs have had to contend with those equally powerful voices of the Flat Earthers of the medical profession who will not accept the work relationship whatever the evidence.

This is not a situation which is likely to continue much longer for there is an increasing acceptance by the medical profession, lawyers, ergonomists and Health & Safety professionals that the relationship between working procedures and upper limb disorders is incontrovertible and developments in research and methodology will ultimately prove this causal relationship.

Chapter 2

# Investigation and Diagnosis

*Abstract – Many past or current medical conditions can confuse or influence the diagnosis of work related upper limb disorders and it is essential that the investigation of WRULDs should include a comprehensive medical and occupational history and physical examination.*

One of the many problems inherent in the diagnosis of WRULDs is the wide spectrum of physical and psychological responses to the same stimulus. These responses not only reflect the obvious individual differences in age, sex, height, weight, work experience and training, but the psychological variation which exists between people, and variations in their physiological and biochemical make up.

For example the young fertile woman can show quite different responses to the same stimuli than would a post menopausal woman. Equally the younger woman will respond differently when she is pre-menstrual or pregnant. This wide biological diversity, and variation on the normal, which exists within homo-sapiens makes it difficult to lay down hard and fast criteria when investigating the many soft tissue changes which are lumped together under the term 'work related upper limb disorder'. Some individuals will happily put up with poor working conditions without any apparent injurious effect to their physical or mental welfare whilst others, exposed to identical working conditions, can suffer a spectrum of health problems ranging from minor muscle aches and pains to total disability.

It is unfortunately impossible however, to tell in advance how an individual will respond to their working conditions.

This variation in response to the same working conditions must be understood when investigating work related upper limb disorders. It must also be born in mind that up to 10% of any industrial workforce will be found on pre-employment medical examination to have a significant medical condition which may influence their working capacity.[21]

Many extraneous factors however, can be excluded if the medical practitioner takes a comprehensive family, social, occupational and medical history with specific questioning on cardio-vascular, respiratory, gastro-intestinal, central-nervous, urino-genital, obstetric, neurological and musculo-skeletal systems – and then follows up any clues brought out in this history.

The history is followed by a comprehensive physical examination where each of the above systems is considered, examined and recorded. Particular care needs to be taken to evaluate the patient's posture and any limitation or abnormalities of upper limb structure and movement. Routine biochemistry, haematology and rheumatology profiles will be carried out. Only in this way is it possible to exclude the many disease processes, genetic factors, and previous traumatic injuries which can interfere with the making of an accurate WRULD diagnosis.

In an increasingly litigious area of medicine, cutting corners in the medical history or physical examination can later lead to embarrassing problems for the medical practitioner.

It would also be desirable to examine the patient's work place, with the patient present and demonstrating working procedures being carried out. In the absence of this, photographs, drawings and written descriptions of working procedures are helpful. When the patient is being examined a demonstration by the patient of the actual upper limb movements being carried out in the working procedures allows a functional analysis of the muscle groups involved and their associated tendons, nerves and blood vessels.

An ergonomics report on the work place can often be very helpful.

Nerve conduction studies are essential for the proper diagnosis of carpal tunnel syndrome and some nerve entrapment conditions. If surgery is contemplated for, say, shoulder impingement or a rotator cuff tear and precise delineation of anatomy is required then CT, arthroscopy, ultra sound, MRI scans and magnetic resonance angiography can all be useful in the right circumstances. Generally speaking plain x-rays of the relevant area are the most useful radiological investigation for WRULDs but when investigating neck and shoulder pain it must be born in mind that degenerative changes in the cervical and thoracic spine are inevitable from early middle age onwards and, by the age of 65, 90% of the UK population have radiological evidence of it. These changes are often unrelated to symptoms and, as they are due to disc/ligamentous changes, undetectable on plain x-ray.

However, the more sophisticated radiological and physiological investigations have generally contributed little to knowledge or diagnosis of WRULDs.

Recent (1997) threshold vibration measurements for peripheral nerves may however, prove of great value.[22]

## Symptoms and Signs of Work Related Upper Limb Disorders

It is possible to say, as a generalisation, that the blue collared workers are more likely to have both signs and symptoms of WRULDs whilst the white collared workers have only symptoms. This crude division whilst useful in diagnosis should be treated with caution.

Not all of the following WRULD symptoms and signs will

be present, nor are they listed in order of precedence, but it is useful for the medical practitioner to have a check list in mind to allow specific questioning of the patient.

Pain
Discomfort
Swelling – real or perceived
Inflammation
Loss of sensation (paraesthesia) (pins and needles)
Loss of muscle bulk
Muscle weakness
Restriction in movement
Crepitus
Loss of fine sensation and the ability to grip small objects.
Ganglion
Tendinitis
Rotator Cuff Injury
Osteoarthritis

It must never be forgotten that each patient is different and the symptoms and signs will vary from one person to another. Nevertheless three stages of progression can be identified based largely on the number of hours the symptoms are present during a 24 hour period.

*(1) Mild*

This is characterised by pain, aching and tiredness in the forearms, hands, wrists, arms shoulders or neck during the working hours. The symptoms improve overnight but return within an hour or so of starting work in the morning. Once established the patient tends to suffer some or all of the symptoms during their working hours and, whilst they continue to do the same work, the symptoms will remain and in time get worse. At this state the symptoms are reversible with a change in the working routines. The patient will often take mild pain killers to mask the symptoms to get through the working day.

*(2) Moderate*

The pain, aching and tiredness in the arms, shoulders and neck persist at night, may disturb sleep, and return very quickly at work in the morning. Signs such as swelling or discolouration of the skin may become apparent and although the symptoms and signs usually disappear when the patient is on holiday they manifest themselves again soon after a return to work. Signs and symptoms may persist for many months, even when the provoking activities have been given up, and there is a general feeling of fatigue. The use of pain killers is common, understandable, but undesirable.

*(3) Severe*

The pain, aching and weakness in the hands, wrists, forearms, upper arms, shoulders and neck are a permanent feature in the life of the sufferer. Sleep is often disturbed and although the patient may take pain killers and night sedation, insomnia may prevail and the problems make it difficult to continue with work or carry out routine domestic and social activities. The lives of those sufferers with severe work related upper limb disorders is significantly and adversely affected. Treatment often brings little benefit and even if the provoking working activity is given up the symptoms and signs may persist for months or years – or prove irreversible.

*Chapter 3*

# Clinical Anatomy

*Abstract – The accurate diagnosis of work related upper limb disorders is dependent upon a knowledge of the relevant anatomy; an understanding of the nature of the patient's working activities; and the skill to identify the anatomical structures involved in, and being compromised by, those activities.*

Accurate diagnosis of WRULDs is important as a preliminary to treatment but it is particularly important if litigation is contemplated as such vague diagnoses as work related upper limb disorder, overuse syndrome, or 'RSI' will not stand up in Court.

Although in theory all muscle groups and their associated nerves and blood vessels may suffer work related injury, in fact, the majority of injuries are in the soft tissues of the hand, forearm and – to a lesser extent – the shoulder.

For example about 75% of WRULDs identified in assembly line or general factory work involve the tendons of only four muscles: abductor pollicis longus and extensor pollicis brevis, and the two radial extensors at the wrist – extensors carpi radialis longus and brevis.[23]

The brachioradialis and supinator muscles are also commonly involved in work related conditions.

The following does not therefore, attempt to be a detailed account of the anatomy of the upper limbs but emphasises those muscles and structures which are likely to be considered in the investigation and diagnosis of WRULDs and should be seen as the anatomical background to the Clinical Syndromes (see Chapter 5).

The muscles of the upper limb are divisible into six groups:

1. Muscles of the hand.
2. Muscles of the forearm.
3. Muscles of the upper arm.
4. Muscles of the shoulder.
5. Muscles connecting the upper limb with the anterior and lateral thoracic walls.
6. Muscles connecting the upper limb with the vertebral column.[24]

## The Hand

The human hand is remarkable and unique in its complexity of structure and versatility of actions. Its powerful grasping mechanism is matched by an ability to carry out the most finely controlled movements and to perform as the chief tactile organ of the body. Such versatility of function is brought about by the integration of a highly sophisticated structure including skin, bones, tendons, muscles, blood vessels, nerves and sweat glands which – as a functional unit – represents one of the high points of evolutionary achievement.

An outline of the muscles of the hand and forearm are given here as it is necessary for the purpose of an accurate diagnosis of WRULD'S's to be able to analyse those basic movements of the hand and forearm which are involved in the commoner working procedures – and to relate these movements to the main muscle groups which bring them about.

Many of the essential movements involved in working procedures take place at the wrists and involve flexion, extension, pronation and supination in combination with flexion, extension and abduction movements of the fingers and thumb.

Because local trauma followed by infection in the hand is very common in all industrial activities it is also necessary to understand the anatomy of the synovial sheaths of the tendons on the front and back of the hands – and their particular relationships with the flexor retinaculum and the carpal tunnel – as a preliminary to understanding the clinical syndromes which involve the synovial sheaths.

The carpal tunnel is a bony tunnel formed by the anterior surfaces of the carpal bones and covered by the strong fibrous bands of the flexor retinaculum at the wrist. The tunnel contains the flexor tendons of the digits and the median nerve. (See carpal tunnel syndrome.)

The following are the muscles and nerves concerned with the movements of the thumb and fingers:

*(a) Muscles Concerned in the Movements of the Thumb*

| *Movement* | *Muscle* | *Principal Nerve Supply* |
|---|---|---|
| Flexion | Flexor pollicus brevis | Median or ulnar |
| | Flexor pollicis brevis | Anterior interosseous |
| | Opponens pollicis | Median |
| Extension | Extensor pollicis brevis | Posterior interosseous |
| | Extensor pollicis longus | Posterior interosseous |
| | Abductor pollicis longus | Posterior interosseous |
| Abduction | Abductor pollicis longus | Posterior interosseous |
| | Abductor pollicis brevis | Median |
| Adduction | Adductor pollicis | Ulnar |
| | First dorsal interosseous | Ulnar |
| | Extensor pollicis longus | Posterior interosseous |
| | Flexor pollicis longus | Anterior interosseous |
| Opposition | Opponens pollicis | Median |
| | Abductor pollicis brevis | Median |
| | Flexor pollicis brevis | Median or ulnar |
| | Flexor pollicis longus | Anterior interosseous |
| | Adductor pollicis | Ulnar |

### *(b) Metacarpophalangeal Joints*

| *Movement* | *Muscle* | *Principal Nerve Supply* |
|---|---|---|
| Flexion | Flexor pollicis longus<br>Flexor pollicis brevis<br>First palmar interosseous<br>Abductor pollicis brevis | Anterior interosseous<br>Median or ulnar<br>Ulnar<br>Median |
| Extension | Extensor pollicis longus<br>Extensor pollicis brevis | Posterior interosseous<br>Posterior interosseous |
| Abduction | Abductor pollicis brevis | Median |
| Adduction | Adductor pollicis<br>First palmar interosseous | Ulnar<br>Ulnar |

### *(c) Interphalangeal Joint*

| *Movement* | *Muscle* | *Principal Nerve Supply* |
|---|---|---|
| Flexion | Flexor pollicis longus | Anterior interosseous |
| Extension | Extensor pollicis longus<br>Abductor pollicis brevis<br>Adductor pollicis<br>Extensor pollicis brevis<br>(occasional insertion) | Posterior interosseous<br>Median<br>Ulnar<br>Posterior interosseous |

The following is a summary of the actions of the muscles of the hand and their relative nerve supply. The muscles for convenience being divided into three groups.

1. The muscles of the thumb which occupy the lateral side of the hand as the thenar eminence.
2. The muscles of the little finger which occupy the medial side of the hand as the hypothenar eminence.
3. The muscles in the middle of the palm and between the metacarpal bones.

*Summary of Action of Muscles in the Hand*

| *Joint(s)* | *Muscle(s)* | *Action* | *Nerve Supply* |
|---|---|---|---|
| MCP 1 | Thenar Group | Opposes thumb – flexes, abducts and rotates it medially acting at the carpo-metacarpal and metacarpophalangeal joints | Median |
| | Adductor pollicis | Adduction | Ulnar |
| | Extensors pollicis longus and brevis | Extension | Radial |
| MCP 2–5 | Two lumbricals and interossei | Flexion | Ulnar |
| | Lateral two lumbricals | Flexion | Median |
| | Extensors digiti communis, indicis and digiti minimi | Extension | Radial |
| | Interossei | Abduction and adduction Ulnar | Ulnar |
| IP1 | Flexor pollicus longus | Flexion | Median |
| | Extensor pollicus longus | Extension | Radial |
| PIP and DIP 2–5 | Two lumbricals and interossei | Extension | Ulnar |

## Posterior Muscles of the Forearm

These extensors are for convenience divided into superficial and deep. The Superficial Group of Muscles are:

- Brachioradialis
- Extensor Carpi Radialis Longus
- Extensor Carpi Radialis Brevis

- Extensor Digitorum
- Extensor Digit Minimi
- Extensor Carpi Ulnaris

*Brachioradialis*

This is the most superficial muscle on the radial (outer) side of the forearm and forms the lateral (inner) border of the cubital fossa. It stands out prominently when the semi-pronated forearm is flexed against resistance as in many lifting movements or in pulling mechanical levers where the forearm is in the mid prone position.

Tenderness over the Brachioradialis would suggest the repetitive movements which produce an overuse syndrome as being due to elbow, not wrist, extension.

*Extensor Carpi Radialis Longus*

This arises mainly from the lower third of the supra condylar ridge of the humerus but it also receives fibres from the common tendon of origin in company with the other four extensor muscles. Although this makes it vulnerable to tennis elbow type conditions, its attachment to the shaft of the humerus provides some protection. For much of its course in the forearm the muscle is a flat tendon which passes over the back of the wrist to insert into the second metacarpal bone. The muscle acts synergically with the flexors of the fingers, and in association with the other extensors, in extending the wrist and abducting the hand. Typists, VDU operators and many assembly line workers are thus at risk from developing pathological changes in the tendon.

*Extensor Carpi Radialis Brevis*

This arises from the lateral epicondyle of the humerus by a tendon common to it and the following three extensor muscles. The common extensor tendon is the site of much work, and non work, related pathology manifesting itself as epicondylitis often called tennis elbow, many industrial handling activities involving repetitive movements of the hands, wrists, and forearms such as small parts assembly, meat and poultry processing and work in potteries, are incriminated, but so is playing musical instruments – and javelin, discus and hammer throwing.

*Extensor Digitorum*

This muscle arises partially from the lateral epicondyle of the humerus by the common tendon and divides into four tendons which pass into the back of the hand and proceeds each to its own digit.

The extensor digitorum extends the fingers at the metacarpophalangeal and interphalangeal joints in opening the hand and relaxing the grip. It also assists in extending the wrist. This muscle is involved in many of the movements of the hand on the assembly line or in other industrial situations but also in writing and using keyboards. Its tendons and their synovial sheaths are vulnerable to repetitive movements and can be the site of tenosynovitis and tendonitis.

*Extensor Digiti Minimi*

This slender muscle has a similar origin at the common extensor tendon to extensor digitorum which it accompanies in the forearm before passing over the back of the hand to the little finger. It extends the fifth finger and has similar functions and vulnerabilities to the extensor digitorum.

*Extensor Carpi Ulnaris*

This robust muscle arises, partially from the lateral epicondyle of the humerus by the common extensor tendon and its tendon is inserted in to the base of the fifth metacarpal bone. In association with the extensors carpi radialis, longus and brevis it acts synergically with the flexors of the fingers in order to steady the wrist when objects are being gripped or when the fist is being clenched. It also helps to extend the wrist and abduct the hand and is thus important, and vulnerable, in many commercial, industrial and social activities.

## The Deep Group Muscles of the Forearm

- Supinator
- Abductor pollicis longus
- Extensor pollicis longus
- Extensor pollicis brevis
- Extensor indicis

*The Supinator*

This surrounds the upper third of the radius and consists of a superficial and a deep part, between which passes the posterior interosseous nerve. The muscle has about six points of origin, including the lateral epicondyle of the humerus, and is inserted into the lateral surface of the proximal third of the radius. It thus rotates the radius so as to turn the palm of the hand forward. Tenderness over the supinator and pain on resisted supination is common in work related upper limb disorders and local swelling may cause compression of the posterior interosseous nerve.

(The word pollicis arises from 'pollex' which is Latin for thumb. Muscles and tendons which control the thumb are a common area of work related pathology.)

*Abductor Pollicis Longus*

This arises from the posterior shafts of both radius and ulna and its tendon is inserted into the base of the first metacarpal bone. Acting with abductor pollicis brevis it abducts the thumb, and acting with the extensors-pollicis, it extends the thumb.

The thumb, particularly the base, is the subject of many complaints of tenderness and chronic pain particularly from those who work in the manufacturing industry where there is great emphasis on manual dexterity. Keyboard work also can be very demanding on the muscles of the thumb.

*Extensor Pollicis Brevis*

This is closely allied in structure and function to the abductor pollicis longus – which extends and rotates the thumb.

The movements of the thumb are complex involving a number of muscles all of which are vulnerable to overuse in the industrial and commercial workplace. Tenosynovitis and crepitation are common findings in the sheaths of the relative tendons. The peculiar sensitivity of the extensor muscles of the wrists and fingers to working conditions has been recognised for centuries. In the nineteenth century paralysis of the extensors leading to 'wrist drop' was common in painters due to lead poisoning. The different muscle groups were effected differently some being capable of recovering whilst others were permanently paralysed. This apparently selective action of the lead in cases of lead poisoning depended in reality upon occupational overuse of the affected muscles or groups of muscles: a phenomena which can still be seen today in keyboard operators or certain workers in the ceramics industry.

*Extensor Indicis*

This is a narrow elongated muscle arising from the posterior shaft of the ulna and passing down the forearm into the wrist and so on to the index finger.

**The Anterior Muscle of the Forearm Superficial Group**

- Pronator teres
- Flexor carpi radialis
- Palmaris longus
- Flexor carpi ulnaris
- Flexor digitorum sublimis

The muscles of this group largely take origin from the medial epicondyle of the humerus by a common tendon which, thus, becomes vulnerable to trauma or pathology in the five associated muscles. Medial epicondylitis is a common element in work related upper limb disorders and is sometimes, but rarely accurately, named 'golfer's elbow'. It is a condition well recognised in javelin throwers and has often been the limiting factor in many a javelin thrower's career (although the triceps muscle is also at risk).

*Pronator Teres*

This muscle has humeral and ulnar heads of origin with the median nerve entering the forearm between those heads. It proceeds from the medial epicondyle to the midpoint of the radius and is prominent when elbow flexion is resisted with the forearm in the mid-prone position. Work related inflammation or hypertrophy of the muscle may compress the median nerve. The pronator teres rotates the radius on the ulna, turning the palm of the hand backwards. Many industrial processes involve the worker in constantly repeated pronation/supination movements and over-use problems in the relevant muscle groups are very common.

*Flexor Carpi Radialis*

This arises largely from the medial epicondyle by the common tendon and its fleshy belly is a prominent part of the forearm until about mid way. It ends in a long tendon which passes under the flexor retinaculum to be inserted into the base of the second metacarpal bone. Flexor carpi radialis acting with flexor carpi ulnaris flexes the wrist and, with the radial extensors, helps to abduct the hand. Constantly repeated flexion and extension movements at the wrist as seen in many types of industrial and commercial activities can create tenosynovitis in the relevant tendon sheaths and this may in turn put pressure on the median nerve where it passes through the carpal tunnel causing carpal tunnel syndrome.

*Palmaris Longus*

This arises as part of the common tendon and may be involved with flexing the wrist. (It is subject to much anatomical variation.)

*Flexor Carpi Ulnaris*

This arises by two heads, humeral and ulnar, beneath which the ulnar nerve takes its vulnerable course downwards, and an artery upwards.

The muscle becomes tendon half way down the forearm, does not pass under the flexor retinaculum, and is inserted into the pisiform bone.

Amongst its other functions flexor carpi ulnaris is one of the powerful flexors of the wrist and abductor of the hand.

*Flexor Digitorum Sublimis*

This is the largest of the muscles of the superficial group and arises by two heads: humero-ulnar and radial. The muscle separates into four tendons which pass beneath the flexor retinaculum to become flexors of the ring, index and little fingers. Because of its bulk and position this muscle can, if swollen, put pressure on the median nerve in the carpal tunnel and thus bring about the carpal tunnel syndrome.

**The Deep Group of Flexors**

- Flexor Digitorum Profundis
- Flexor Pollicis Longus
- Pronator Quadratus

*Flexor Digitorum Profundis*

This arises largely from the shaft of the ulnar and ends in four long tendons which pass beneath the flexor retinaculum and are inserted into the palmar surfaces of the bases of the distal phalanges of the index, middle, ring and little fingers. The muscle flexes the tips of the fingers and assists in flexing the wrist.

The tendons of the flexor digitorum profundis in the

fingers lie in canals lined by synovial sheath which is reflected onto the contained tendon. The relationship between these sheaths and those of flexor digitorum sublimis can have important implications in work related upper limb disorders (see carpal tunnel syndrome).

*Flexor Pollicis Longus*
This arises largely from the shaft of the radius and its tendon, which passes beneath the flexor retinaculum, is inserted into the palmar surface of the base of the distal phalanx of the thumb and its action is to flex the phalanges of the thumb.

The flexor pollicis longus has its own synovial sheath, similar to those for the flexor tendons of the fingers. This can have profound significance from the point of work related upper limb disorders for this sheath extends into the forearm for about 2.5 cm above the flexor retinaculum and may even communicate with other synovial sheaths.

*Pronator Quadratus*
This is a weak pronator and has other functions.

## Movements at the Wrist

Movements of the wrist take place at the radiocarpal and midcarpal joints. The radiocarpal joint is more concerned in extension and adduction at the wrist than the midcarpal, which is responsible for the greater part of flexion and abduction.

*Muscles Concerned in the Movements at the Radiocarpal and Midcarpal Joints*

| *Movement* | *Muscle* | *Principal Nerve Supply* |
|---|---|---|
| Flexion | Flexor carpi radialis | Median |
| | Flexor carpi ulnaris | Ulnar |
| | Palmaris longus | Median |

| | | |
|---|---|---|
| | Flexor digitorum profundus | Anterior interosseous:ulnar |
| | Flexor digitorum superficialis | Median |
| | Flexor pollicis longus | Anterior interosseous |
| | Abductor pollicis longus | Posterior interosseous |
| | Extensor pollicis brevis | Posterior interosseous |
| Extension | Extensor carpi radialis longus | Radial |
| | Extensor carpi radialis brevis | Radial |
| | Extensor carpi ulnaris | Posterior interosseous |
| | Extensor digitorum | Posterior interosseous |
| | Extensor pollicis longus | Posterior interosseous |
| | Extensor indicis | Posterior interosseous |
| | Extensor digiti minimi | Posterior interosseous |
| Abduction | Extensor carpi radialis longus | Radial |
| | Extensor carpi radialis brevis | Radial |
| | Flexor carpi radialis | Median |
| | Abductor pollicis longus | Posterior interosseous |
| | Extensor pollicis brevis | Posterior interosseous |
| | Extensor pollicis longus | Posterior interosseous |
| Adduction | Flexor carpi ulnaris | Ulnar |
| | Extensor carpi ulnaris | Posterior interosseous |

## Movements of the Radio-Ulnar Joints

The two strong supinators are biceps and supinator. The chief pronators are pronator quadratus and pronator teres, but flexor carpi radialis, which passes obliquely from medial to lateral side in the front of the forearm, is capable of assisting. Both supination and pronation are most powerful when the elbow is flexed to a right angle.

*Muscles Concerned in Movements at the Radio-Ulnar Joints*

| *Movement* | *Muscle* | *Principal Nerve Supply* |
|---|---|---|
| Supination | Supinator | Radial |
| | Biceps brachii | Musculocutaneous |
| Pronation | Pronator quadratus | Anterior interosseous |
| | Pronator teres | Median |
| | Flexor Carpi radialis | Median |

## Movements at the Elbow

These movements are considerably influenced by gravity. From the anatomical position the elbow can be flexed and then extended by the flexors alone, even though the triceps and anconeus are paralysed. Again a patient with paralysed flexors can both flex and extend the elbow by the triceps alone if the upper limb is raised above the head.

The more important of the two movements is flexion, which depends on several groups of muscles. Some of the muscles are not normally used to flex the elbow, but can assist in the movement in case of difficulty, particularly pronator teres and flexor carpi radialis. Flexion has thus the safeguard of being mediated by three nerves – musculocutaneous, radial and median, whereas extension depends on one nerve alone, the radialis.

*Muscles Concerned in Movements at the Elbow Joint*

| *Movement* | *Muscle* | *Principal Nerve Supply* |
|---|---|---|
| Flexion | Brachialis | Musculocutaneous |
| | Biceps brachii | Musculocutaneous |
| | Brachioradialis | Radial |
| | Extensor carpi radialis longus | Radial |
| | Pronator teres | Median |
| | Flexor carpi radialis | Median |
| Extension | Triceps brachii | Radial |
| | Anconeus | Radial |

## The Shoulder

The shoulder 'joint' comprises of three components:

1. The gleno-humeral joint (or shoulder joint proper).
2. The acromio-clavicular joint.
3. The sterno-clavicular joint.

The gleno-humeral joint allows a free range of abduction, flexion and rotation under the control of the scapula-humeral muscles.

## The muscles connecting the upper limb with the vertebral column

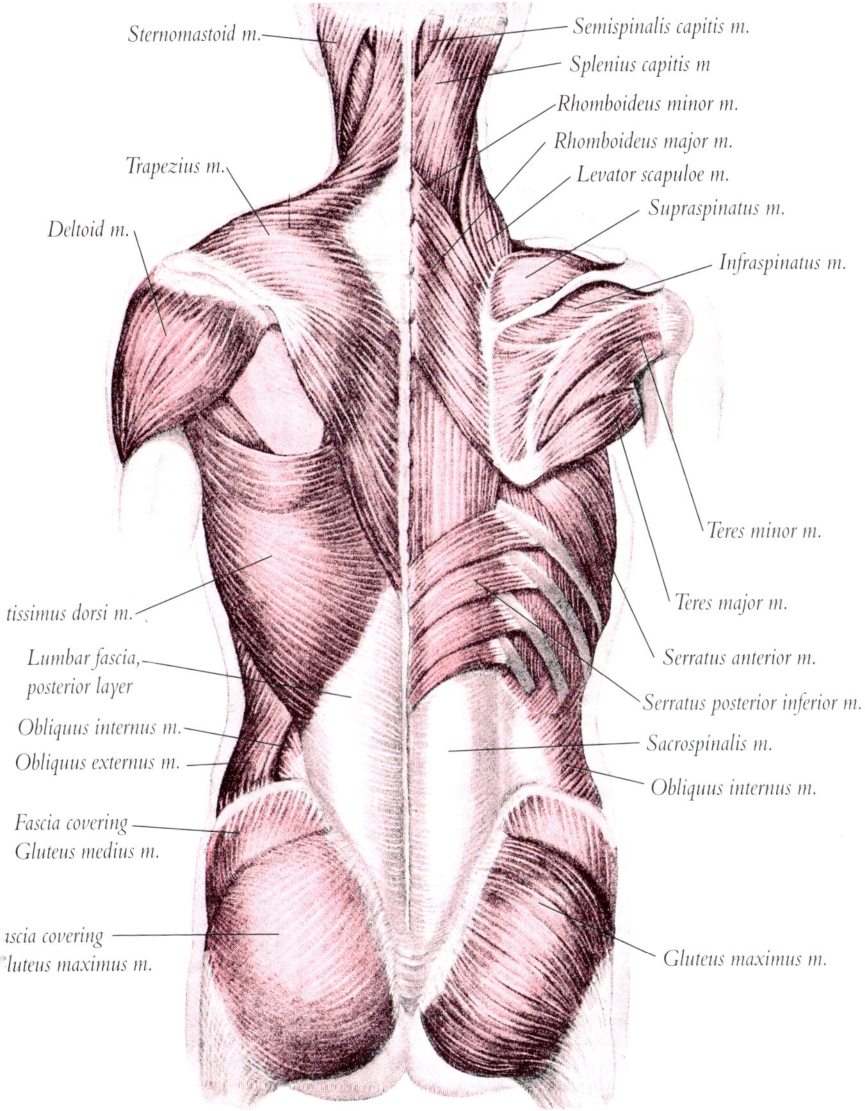

## The superficial flexor muscles of the left forearm

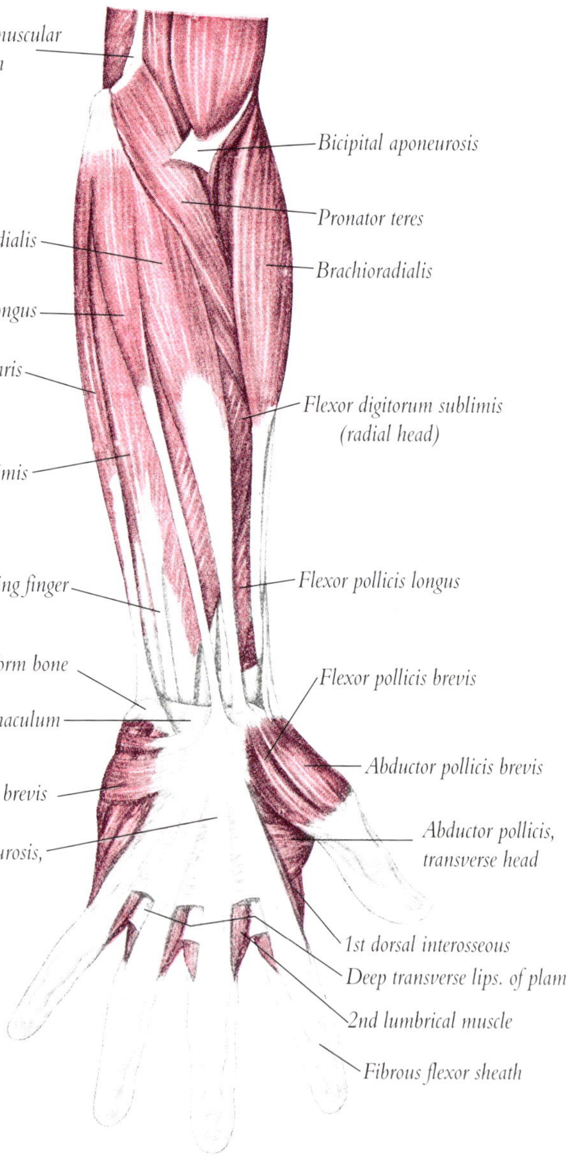

The deep flexor muscles of the forearm

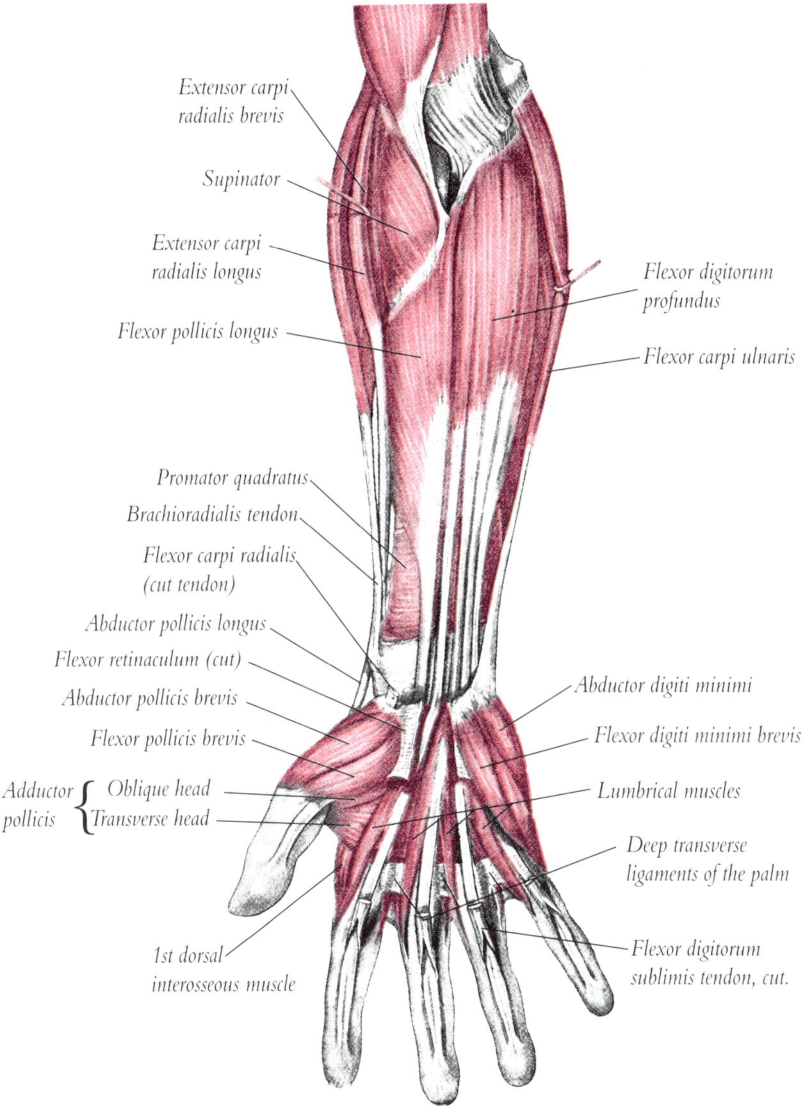

The superficial extensor muscles of the forearm

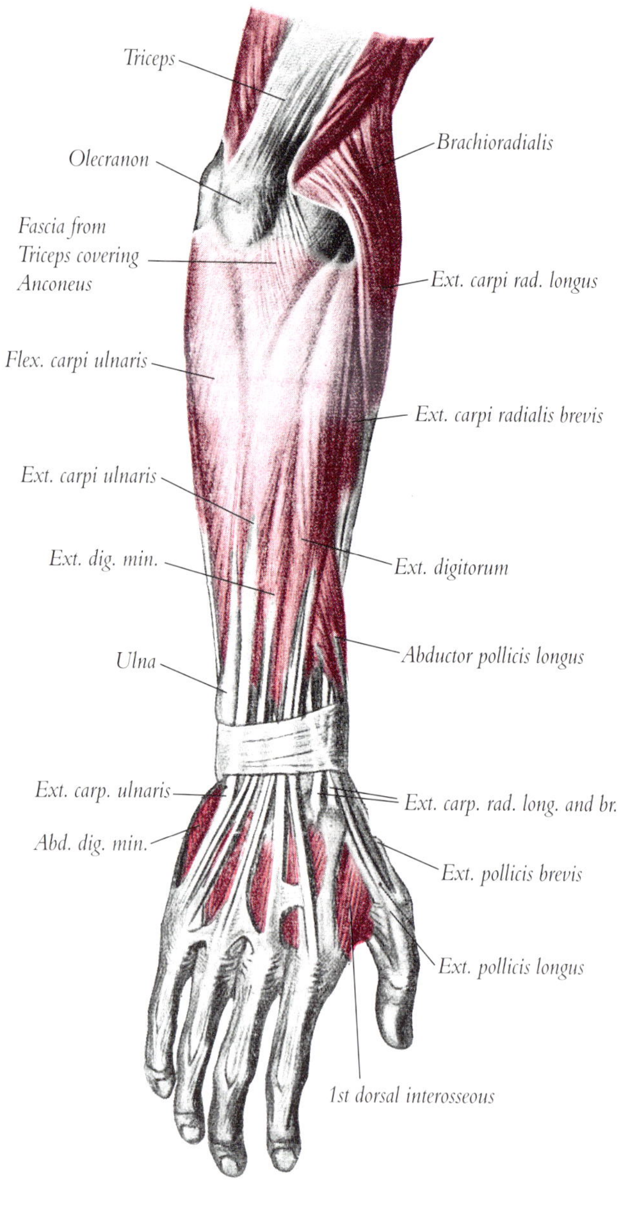

# The deep extensor muscles of the forearm

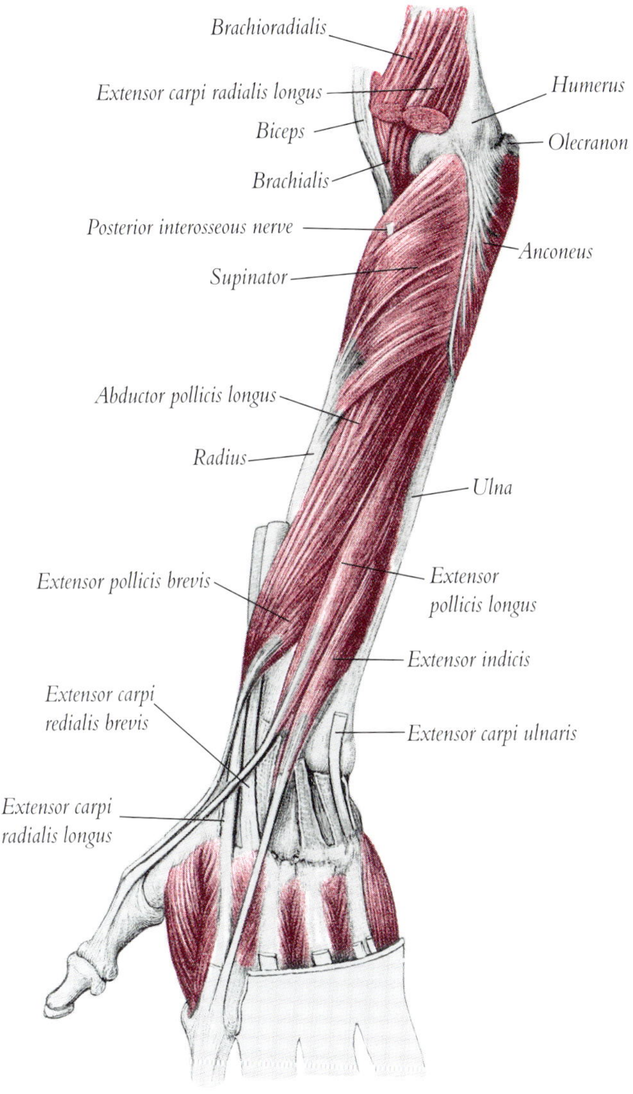

Section through the left carpal tunnel

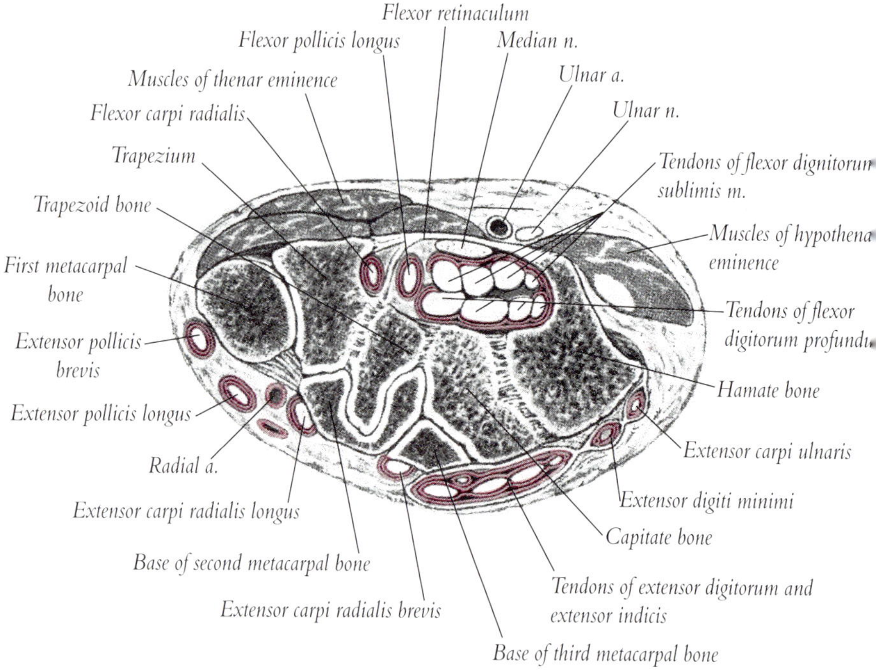

Aspects of the right elbow

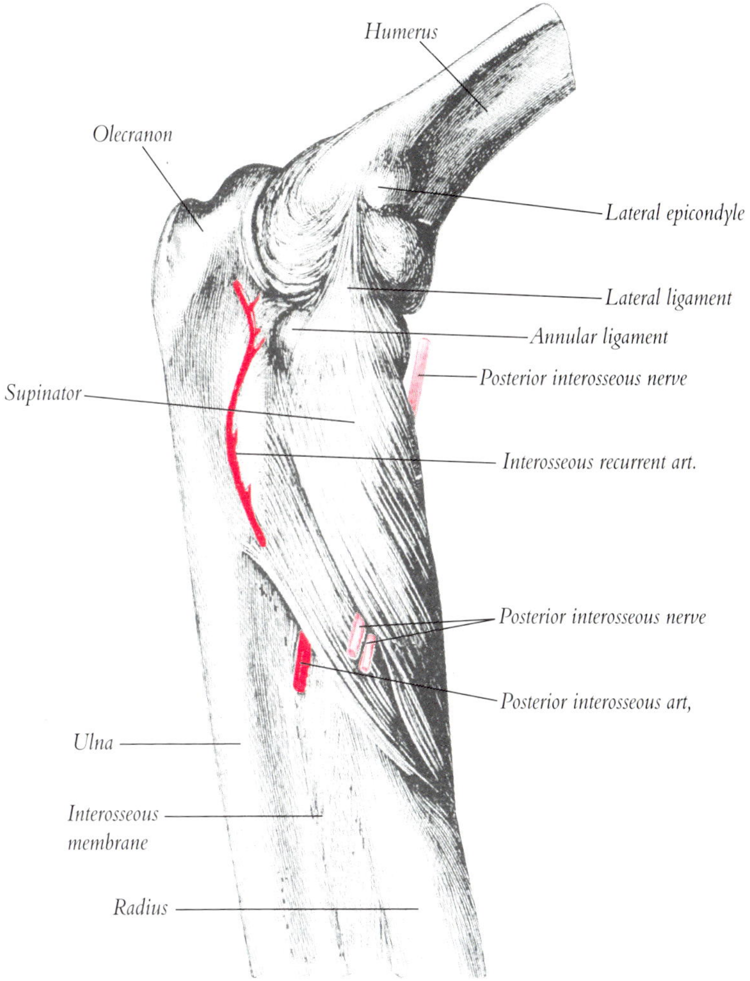

The synovial sheaths of the tendons on the front of the left wrist and hand

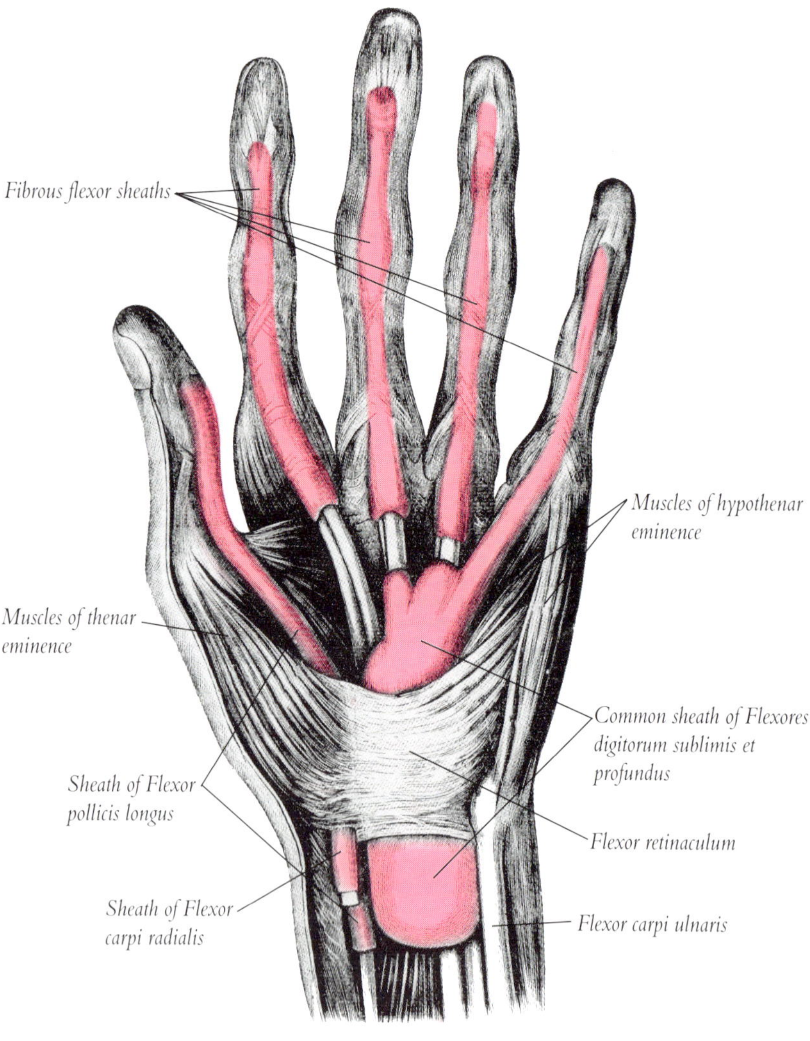

The other two joints together allow 90 degree of rotation of the scapular upon the thorax and a moderate range of anterior-posterior gliding movements of the scapula under the control of the cervico-scapular and thoraco-scapular muscles.

There are many causes of pain in or around the shoulder joint and it is important to be accurate in diagnosis so as to identify those conditions which will respond to treatment.

Causes are:

Rotator cuff tendinitis (subscapularis, infraspinatus)
Supraspinatus tendinitis which may be due to calcium deposits
Adhesive capsulitis (frozen shoulder)
Subacromial bursitis
Bicipital tendinitis (long head of the biceps)
Osteoarthritis of the acromioclavicular joint
Rheumatoid arthritis.

Glenohumeral instability is most likely in the under 25 year olds, tendinitis (impingement) in the 25 to 40 year old age group, and adhesive capsulitis in the over 40 year old age group with a higher incidence in diabetics. Generally however, shoulder pain occurs most commonly in the middle aged or older age group and the incidence appears to plateau at about 45 years of age. Women are affected more frequently than men.

Most WRULDs involving the shoulder are caused by soft tissue lesions affecting the rotator cuff. These painful lesions occur in tendons or tenoperiosteal junctions. They are naturally tender on palpation or create pain on active or resisted movements of the affected part. Osteoarthritis and inflammatory arthritis are less common causes. Osteoarthritis practically never affects the shoulder joint but commonly affects the acromioclavicular joint in the over 50 year old patient.

Lesions of any or all the tendons of the rotator cuff may be caused by repetitive or acute occupational strain. Acute strain of the supraspinatus tendon occurs commonly in work related or sports injuries. Bicipital tendinitis, a form of tenosynovitis affects the tendon sheaths of the long head of the biceps. Frozen shoulder is the most chronic of shoulder conditions and indicates strain of all the rotator cuff tendons, causing a capsulitis.

True shoulder pain is seldom confined to the shoulder itself. Typically it radiates from a point near the tip of the acromion down the lateral side of the upper arm to about the level of the deltoid insertion. It is unusual for pain originating in the shoulder to extend down below the elbow.

Pain arising in the acromio-clavicular joint or sterno-clavicular is localised to the joint itself and does not radiate down the arm.

Pain may be referred to the shoulder from the brachial plexus but unlike true shoulder pain it may radiate down the arm to the hand as 'pins and needles' or 'a numb feeling'.

Repetitive industrial activities involving the arms and shoulder, or specific activities such as plastering ceilings, or the working procedures carried out above the head where the arms are abducted/raised for long periods, such as placing poultry carcasses on to a moving hook line, put unacceptable stresses on the shoulder joints.

*Muscles Concerned in the Movements of the Shoulder Joint.*

| *Movement* | *Muscle* | *Principal Nerve Supply* |
|---|---|---|
| Flexion | Deltoid (anterior portion) | Axillary |
| | Pectoralis major (clavicular portion:sternocostal portion flexes the extended humerus as far as the position of rest) Coracobrachialis. Biceps brachii | Medial and lateral pectoral |
| | | Musculocutaneous |
| | | Musculocutaneous |

| *Movement* | *Muscle* | *Principal Nerve Supply* |
|---|---|---|
| Extension | Deltoid (posterior portion)<br>Teres major (of flexed humerus)<br>Latissimus dorsi (of flexed humerus)<br>Sternocostal portion off pectoralis major<br>(of flexed humerus)<br>Long head of triceps (to position of rest) | Axillary<br><br>Lower subscapular<br>Thoracodorsal<br><br>Medial and pectoral<br>Radial |
| Abduction | Deltoid (middle portion)<br>Supraspinatus<br>Biceps brachii (long head) | Axillary<br>Suprascapular<br>Musculocutaneous |
| Adduction | Pectoralis major<br><br>Latissimus dorsi Teres major<br>Triceps (long head)<br>Coracobrachialis | Medial and lateral pectoral<br>Thoracodorsal<br>Lower subscapular<br>Radial<br>Musculocutaneous |
| Lateral rotation | Deltoid (posterior portion)<br>Infraspinatus<br>Teres minor | Axillary<br>Suprascapular<br>Axillary |
| Medial rotations | Pectoralis major<br><br>Teres major<br>Latissimus dorsi<br>Deltoid (anterior portion)<br>Subscapularis | Medial and lateral pectoral<br>Lower subscapular<br>Thoracodorsal<br>Axillary<br><br>Upper and lower subscapular |
| Horizontal flexion | Deltoid (anterior portion)<br>Pectoralis major<br>Subscapularis | Axillary<br>Medial and lateral pectoral<br>Upper and lower subscapular |
| Horizontal extension | Deltoid (posterior portion)<br>Infraspinatus | Axillary<br>Suprascapular |

## Muscles Connecting the Upper Limb with the Vertebral Column

Degenerative changes in the cervical spine (cervical spondylosis) are the commonest orthopaedic cause of neck disorders.[25] This may lead to interference with the roots of the brachial plexus causing radiating pain, muscle weakness or sensory impairment in the upper limb and pins and needles and numbness in the hands. Thus the clinical importance of cervical spondylosis may often be in its neurological effects rather than in the actual local degenerative changes.

Ergonomically unsound working conditions, as such, are an unusual cause of WRULDs although they may well exacerbate existing degenerative changes in the neck or back.

Long periods with the neck flexed looking at a VDU certainly cause neck stiffness and a poor working posture – perhaps due to badly designed chairs or work stations – will, if persisted with for long periods without breaks, lead to chronic aches and pains in the neck.[26,27] Whether they are the cause of degenerative changes in the cervical spine is a moot point. In the opinion of the author poor posture merely exacerbates a pre-existing condition which is commonly present as part of the natural ageing process or may be secondary to whiplash trauma.

The same will apply to local aches and pains in the trapezius muscles, and other muscles which impinge on the vertebral column.

*Muscles Concerned in the Movements of the Shoulder Girdle*

| *Movement* | *Muscle* | *Principal Nerve Supply* |
|---|---|---|
| Elevation | Trapezius (upper fibres) | Spinal part of accessory |
| | Levator scapulae | Ventral rami of C.3, 4, 5 |
| | Rhomboideus major | Ventral ramus of C.5 |
| | Rhomboideus minor | Ventral; ramus of C.5 |
| | Sternocleidomastoid | Spinal part of accessory |

| *Movement* | *Muscle* | *Principal Nerve Supply* |
|---|---|---|
| Depression | Trapezius (lower fibres)<br>Pectoralis minor<br>Pectoralis major (sternocostal portion)<br>Latissimus dorsi | Spinal part of accessory<br>Medial and lateral pectoral<br>Medial and lateral pectoral<br><br>Thoracodorsal |
| Protraction | Serratus anterior<br>Pectoralis minor<br>Pectoralis major | Long thoracic<br>Medial and lateral pectoral<br>Medial and lateral pectoral |
| Retraction | Trapezius (middle fibres)<br>Rhomboideus major<br>Rhomboideus minor<br>Latissimus dorsi | Spinal part of accessory<br>Ventral ramus of C.5<br>Ventral ramus of C.5<br>Thoracodorsal |
| Lateral displacement of inferior angle of scapula | Serratus anterior<br>Trapezius (upper and lower fibres) | Long thoracic<br>Spinal part of accessory |
| Medial displacement of inferior angle of scapula | Pectoralis minor<br>Rhomboideus major<br>Rhomboideus minor<br>Latissimus dorsi | Medial and lateral pectoral<br>Ventral ramus of C.5<br>Ventral ramus of C.5<br>Thoracodorsal |

*Chapter 4*

# The Clinical Syndromes

*Abstract – Thirteen upper limb conditions are described in terms of their anatomical structure, signs, symptoms, diagnosis and treatment. The non specific pain syndrome is also discussed. Between them they cover the whole spectrum of WRULDs's.*

There is no definite list of what constitutes WRULDs and different authorities have differing views on what should be included or excluded from the list of clinical syndromes.

Some authorities consider that reflex sympathetic dystrophy should be included in this section as a clinical syndrome in its own right. I have taken the view that the condition is more likely to be a secondary complication of upper limb disorders than a primary cause of them. I have also included sheath infections for, whilst not primarily a musculo-skeletal condition, they are commonly work related and can lead to soft tissue involvement.

## *(a)* Carpal Tunnel Syndrome

This is a common cause of discomfort in the hand, especially in middle aged or elderly women. It is caused by pressure on the median nerve as it passes within the firm walled carpal tunnel from the forearm into the hand. The pressure produces a tingling numbness or discomfort in the radial (outer) three and a half fingers and there is a feeling of clumsiness in carrying out fine movements such as those involved in sewing. The symptoms and signs vary with the degree and duration of the compression of the median nerve but include weakness or wasting of the abductor pollicis brevis muscle, sensory loss and exacerbation of symptoms at night.

Carpal tunnel syndrome is confirmed by abnormal nerve conduction tests and positive Phelan's and Tinel's tests. When properly diagnosed the results of surgery are good.[26•27•28]

It is thought that repeated flexion and extension at the wrist, as in various work related activities, can cause fluid to accumulate and put pressure on the median nerve causing the typical carpal tunnel syndrome. A number of reports have detailed the changing anatomic relationship between median nerve and finger flexor tendons during flexion and extension. When the wrist is in the neutral position, tension on finger flexor tendons remains restricted to the tendons themselves. Wrist flexion compresses the median nerve between the flexor tendons and flexor retinaculum. With wrist extension, the nerve is stretched over the flexor tendons and head of the radius bone.[29•30•31] Magnetic resonance imaging (MRI) studies of carpal tunnel dimensions during wrist flexion demonstrate a reduction in available space between median nerve, flexor tendons, and retinaculum.[32] Smith and associates show how the median nerve was subjected to the greatest compression when the flexor profundus tendons of the second and third fingers were subjected to force while the wrist was flexed.

Wrist flexion and extension have been associated with changes in intracanal pressure recordings. Brian and associates[33] reported that pressure within the carpal tunnel were increased by 100 mm Hg with wrist flexion and 300 mm Hg with wrist extension. Patients with carpal tunnel syndrome have long been suspected of having increased carpal tunnel pressure at rest, somewhere about 30 mm Hg, with normal being 7 to 8 mm HG.[31•34•35] It was postulated that these changes, over time, could result in a cycle of progressive nerve edema and ischemia.[34•35] In patients with carpal tunnel syndrome, not only is canal pressure above normal at rest but once elevated by wrist movement, pressures continue to remain high, in contrast to what occurs in normal individuals. The underlying cause of the increased canal pressure is not clear but may be a consequence of chronic edema and fibrosis of the flexor tendon synovium.[36]

It has been suggested that repetitive hand and wrist activity has been to promote synovial edema and fibrosis, leading to elevated carpal tunnel pressure. Intermittent pressure rises may occur during wrist flexion and extension, possibly creating a damaging cycle of edema, rising pressure, vascular compromise, and eventually nerve compression.[36] There are however, other causes of neurological disturbances in the hand including those arising in the neck, from interference with the brachial plexus, and lesions of the median nerve elsewhere in its anatomical course. Such diseases as muscular dystrophy and syringomyelia may also cause similar neurological disturbance and must be excluded.

The condition may also be caused by weight increase or fluid retention such as in pregnancy – it is also more common amongst women taking the contraceptive pill.

Collagen disorders, osteoarthritis and previous trauma affecting the bones of the wrist joint should also be excluded. Also myxoedema or frank obesity.

Surveys suggest 20,000 work related carpal tunnel syndromes a year in the UK which is probably a conservative estimate.[21]

Feldman et al and Birkbeck and Beer have shown the relationships between carpal tunnel syndromes and various working activities.[37•38]

The Industrial Injuries Advisory Council (IIAC) reporting on work related upper limb disorders in 1992 stated that:

'from overwhelming clinical evidence we believe

> that many other cases of carpal tunnel syndrome (besides the use of hand held vibrating tools) are also occupationally caused and that this can be proven on an individual basis by clinical tests. We are therefore, recommending that, exceptionally, carpal tunnel syndrome should be prescribed'

This recommendation has not so far been implemented.

*(b)* **Tenosynovitis**

*Teno*: refers to tendon.
*Synov*: refers to the thin covering of membrane.
*Itis*: means inflammation.

Tenosynovitis is thus inflammation of the thin synovial lining of a tendon sheath and, the term should not be used when the tenosynovium is normal or absent. Where there is excessive friction from overuse the synovial sheath is mildly inflamed and there is an exudate of watery fluid within it. This may be associated with pain, crepitus, tenderness and swelling.

The most affected tendons are the long radial extensors of the fingers at the wrist and the abductors of the thumb.[23]

Peritendinitis crepitus occurs at the musculotendinous junction above the upper limit of the tendon sheath in the forearm and, whilst distinct from tenosynovitis – though prescribed – they have much in common: pain on resisted movement, swelling, tenderness and crepitus.

In a study of motor vehicle assembly plant workers the main etiological factors were occupational change necessitating unaccustomed movements, resumption of work after absence, and repetitive stereotype movements.[23]

Although tenosynovitis is a clear cut entity, the term is often applied to situations in which there is no synovia and only vague aches and pains in the wrists and forearms. Such diagnoses are unhelpful – particularly if litigation is contemplated. Often before any specific diagnostic signs are present the factory doctor or general practitioner writes 'tenosynovitis' on the sick note. This initial misdiagnosis of tenosynovitis is a frequent source of misunderstanding and may start the patient on the course towards litigation Hence the reason to make an accurate diagnosis in the first place.

In Britain since 1947 tenosynovitis has been a prescribed disease (A8) and is the second most frequent cause of certified incapacity to work – after occupational dermatitis. The DSS lists it as:

> 'Traumatic inflammation of the tendons of the hand or forearm, or of the associated tendon sheaths'

and lists the type of job likely to cause it as:

> 'Manual labour of frequent or repeated movements of the hand or wrist. For example, manual assembly worker'

### *(c)* Epicondylitis

This is characterised by pain in the lateral or medial aspect of the elbow joint which often radiates down into the forearm. It is due to some form of lesion, which may include inflammation or tearing, caused by strain on the forearm extensor or flexor muscles at their point of origin.

It occurs in occupations in which there are active or resisted movements of the forearm muscles as, for example, in the use of screwdrivers or other hand held tools.

Epicondylitis appears under many names – all unsatisfactory – such as tennis elbow, golfer's elbow, javelin thrower's arm, but many occupational activities involving hammering or lifting with outstretched fingers may bring about this typical clinical picture. It is often difficult to decide whether the condition is work related and needs to be differentiated from local nerve entrapment and referred shoulder and neck pain.

Acute tennis elbow is common in young to middle aged patients as a result of strain of the extensor tendons of the forearm at the tenoperiosteal insertion into the extensor epicondyle of the humerus. On palpation there is exquisite pain and localised tenderness over the lateral epicondyle of the humerus. The pain may be reproduced by asking the patient to extend the hand at the wrist (dorsi flexion) against resistance. All other movements at the elbow are normal.

The common insertion of the extensor muscles of the forearm and the hand is made up of brachioradialis, extensor carpi radialis, extensor carpi ulnaris and the digitorum muscles. Strain of any of these muscles at their insertion will cause a tendonitis at this site, which will produce an easily localised point of acute tenderness.

When carrying out a local injection using steroid alone is more painful for the patient, but the overall success of the injection is higher because the operator will be able to detect all the painful parts of the lesion which is impossible if a local anaesthetic is also used. Success depends on identifying and infiltrating all the points of tenderness in the tenoperiosteal junction at one injection.

Golfer's elbow mirrors the lesion of tennis elbow and occur in the origin of the forearm flexor muscles at the medial epicondyle of the humerus. It is also so known as medial epicondylitis and may be caused repetitive movements affecting the flexor muscle group.

The patient complains of acute tenderness on a spot over the medial epicondyle, which is easily reproduced by asking the patient to flex the hand at the wrist against resistance.

The common flexor tendon insertion involves flexor carpi radialis, digitorum superficialis, flexor carpi ulnaris and palmaris longus. As in tennis elbow, the lesion is localised to the tenoperiosteal junction. The ulnar nerve is in close proximity in the canal posterior to the medial epicondyle and may be punctured easily by an injecting needle. Prior to the injection, when the needle is in situ, the doctor should confirm that no paraesthesia are felt in the ulnar distribution, i.e. in the little finger and the ulnar side of the ring finger.

Lateral or medial epicondylitis can manifest itself suddenly and there can be exquisitely tender areas on palpation over the epicondyles particularly when the ulnar nerve passes over the medial epicondyle – ulnar neuritis. It can disappear equally suddenly. Treatment is, on the whole, unsatisfactory and even if the use of local steroid injections are ultimately successful the patient may need to put up with pain for up to 48 hours after the injection.

### *(d)* de Quervain's Stenosing Tenovaginitis

This has been described as a type of tenosynovitis (although the synovial tendon sheath is not inflamed) of the tendons of the muscles of the thumb as they pass into the wrist. The pain is over the styloid process of the radius and there may be a palpable nodule – due to thickening of the fibrous sheath – in the course of the abductor pollicus longus and extensor pollicus brevis tendons. This is a similar condition to trigger finger.

The cause is unknown but is mainly suffered by women and may be associated with repetitive activities involving much use of the thumb, forefinger and wrists such as working at knitting machines, on assembly lines, wringing out washing and switch board operating.

The main symptoms are pain exacerbated by resisted thumb extension and associated with a positive Finkelstein's test. The condition needs to be distinguished from other pathological conditions, such as local osteo-arthritis. If it does not clear up spontaneously local steroid injections or surgical decompression may help.

### *(e)* Shoulder Capsulitis (Frozen Shoulder)

This is characterised by aches and pains in the shoulder and upper arm of gradual or spontaneous onset associated with impairment of active and passive movement. The cause is not understood but is probably related to repetitive use, or misuse, of the shoulder joint which may lead to loss of resilience possibly due to adhesions of the joint capsule.

Complaints of shoulder/neck pain are extremely common in all work situations and are multifactorial. Thus pre-existing disease factors must be excluded.

Arthroscopy and MRI scans may identify a reduction in the synovial cavity with the restriction being in the glenohumeral area. There is restricted external rotation, abduction and internal rotation of the humerus.

A differential diagnosis must be made between the local pain and referred pain from neck, shoulder, pulmonary or the cardio-vascular system. The condition may resolve spontaneously with a return to normal function particularly if treated early on. It can also develop into a chronic condition.

*(f)* **Rotator Cuff Syndrome** (Shoulder Tendonitis)

The rotator cuff refers to a cuff of soft tissue over the tip of the shoulder made up of the supraspinatus tendon and the adjoining flat tendons of the infraspinatus behind, and subcapularis in front which are blended together to form what is often called the rotator cuff. Distally, the tendons forming the cuff blend with the capsule of the shoulder. The tendons of the biceps can also be part of this syndrome.

Lesions of any, or all, of the tendons of the rotator cuff may be caused by many repetitive or active occupational activities.

Injury to the cuff generally produces pain at the tip of the shoulder and down the upper arm to the deltoid muscle, associated with pain on restricted movement, inability to raise the arm and limitation of various other movements of the arm.

It will be apparent that this syndrome may involve the tendons of one or more of five muscles as well as the shoulder capsule and so the clinical findings will vary according to the soft tissue involved.

Acute strain of the supraspinatus tendon may be associated with working activities where arms are elevated above the head. It is diagnosed by abducting both arms palms upwards to 90 degrees. Placing both hands on the back of the head is external rotation and the movement is performed by the infraspinatus muscle and any restriction is due to infraspinatus tendinitis. The subscapularis muscle is investigated by bringing each arm in turn behind the back and raising the thumbs to reach the bra strap or touch the spine. This is internal rotation and any restriction id due to subscapularis tendinitis.

If pain is experienced when the arms are raised from 90 degrees to 180 degrees – horizontal to vertical – this suggests osteoarthritis of the acromioclavicular joint. This movement is performed by the supraspinatus and any restriction is due to tendinitis. Bicipital tendinitis is due to strain of the long heads of the biceps tendon and is a form of tenosynovitis presenting as pain at the tip of the shoulder on resisted supination of the wrist and tenderness on palpation over the bicipital groove. It is related to many working activities but may respond dramatically to steroid injections accurately into the synovial sheath.

### *(g)* Nerve Entrapments

A number of nerves in the upper arm are subject to entrapment.

- Carpal tunnel syndrome involves the median nerve and has been dealt with elsewhere.
- The ulnar nerve is vulnerable at the wrist and the medial epicondyle at the elbow.
- The posterior interosseous nerve possesses its own syndrome called the radial tunnel syndrome.

Radial tunnel syndrome is caused by pressure on the posterior interosseous nerve within the tunnel formed by five anatomical structures at the lateral epicondyle (outer aspect of the elbow) and is the explanation for one of the many causes of pain in the elbow. Diagnostically the pain is worsened if the middle finger is pressed backwards and improved by anaesthetic block within the radial tunnel. The syndrome may be work related and tends to improve with rest. Surgery may help by decompressing the posterior interosseous nerve within the radial tunnel. But it may not. The use of local anti-inflammatory drugs may also be beneficial.

### *(h)* **Thoracic Outlet Syndrome**

The author has doubts about the reality of this as a work related syndrome. It is said to be caused by compression in the root of the neck by anatomically abnormal structures such as cervical rib or fibrous bands and the symptoms depend on whether nerve or blood vessel is constricted. Symptoms may thus be exacerbated by work but is unlikely to be caused by work.

### *(i)* **Vibration White Finger** (Raynaud's Phenomenon of Occupational Origin)

The use of vibrating tools dates from about 1883, with reports of associated symptoms in the hand from the early 1990s This is a condition in which the control of the blood vessels to the fingers is disturbed and one or more of the fingers become white as the blood supply is closed off. The hands become clumsy particularly in cold weather or cold working conditions. It is progressive and irreversible.

The symptoms of intermittent blanching of the fingers can be due to many other causes including a constitutional predisposition, mainly amongst women; disease processes, such as connective tissue diseases; neurogenic disease, such as syringomyelia; vascular disease, such as arteriosclerosis; and trauma, frostbite, smoking and various drugs – all of which must be excluded before the diagnosis of vibration white finger is made.

Vibration white finger has been a prescribed disease since 1985 (A11) and its occurrence in association with certain occupations may give rise to compensation by the government. Workers may also sue their employers in the civil courts. In order to establish the diagnosis there has to be a history of exposure to vibration with the exclusion of other possible causes.

The Department of Social Security is very specific in listing the signs and symptoms of vibration white finger as follows:

> Episodic blanching, occurring throughout the year, affecting the middle or proximal phalanges, or in the case off a thumb the proximal phalanx, of:
>
> (1) In the case of a person with fingers (including thumb) on one hand, any three of those fingers.
>
> or
>
> (2) In the case of a person with only four such fingers, any two of those fingers.
>
> or
>
> (3) In the case of a person with less than four such fingers, any one of those fingers, or as the case may be, the one remaining finger.

The DSS is equally specific when listing the type of tools and machinery:

> (1) The use of hand held chain saws, in forestry.
>
> or
>
> (2) The use of hand held rotary tools in grinding or in the sanding or polishing of metal, or the holding of material being ground, or metal being sanded or polished by rotary tools.
>
> or
>
> (3) The use of hand held percussive metal working tools, or

the holding of metal being worked upon by percussive tools, in rivetting, caulking, chipping, hammering, fettling or swaging.

or

(4) The use of hand held powered percussive drills or hand held powered percussive hammers in mining, quarrying, demolition, or on roads or footpaths, including road construction.

or

(5) The holding of materials being worked upon by pounding machines in shoe manufacture.

There have been some very significant, recent (1997/1998) decisions against British Coal and British Gas – involving thousands of miners and gas workers who had used pneumatic hammers and drills.

### *(j)* Sheath Infections of the Hands

The hands are constantly exposed to injury in many industrial processes and infections of the sheaths of the flexor tendons are common – particularly if gloves are not worn – and can spread rapidly. The extent of the spread of infection depends on the digit involved.

The synovial sheaths of the three middle digits are isolated and infection will thus be limited. The synovial sheaths of the thumb and the little finger however, communicate with the larger synovial sheaths which surround the flexor tendons and inflammation may thus extend into the palm of the hand, and behind the flexor retinaculum, into the forearm.

Chronic inflammation of the common flexor sheaths can occur if the initial inflammation is not treated in its early stages. Infection of the sheath can also extend to local tissue giving rise to a subcutaneous cellulitis of the hand, otherwise known as beat hand – one of the prescribed industrial diseases (A5). This condition is particularly prevalent among workers carrying out heavy manual labour using hand held tools such as spades, shovels and picks. It may also arise from the need to repeatedly strike the palm of the hand on to a hard surface in such procedures as the opening or closing of potato, onion or other agricultural hoppers. The tissues become devitalised by constant bruising making them more vulnerable to infection.

### *(k)* Cramp of the Hand or Forearm

This has the advantage of being a prescribed disease (A4) having been included in the list since 1948 by the Department of Health & Social Security for the purpose of industrial injury benefit. In leaflet N12 issued by the DHSS in 1983 it is described as:

> 'Cramp of the hand or forearm due to the repetitive movements; e.g. Writer's cramp. Type of occupations includes any occupation involving prolonged periods of handwriting, typing, or other repetitive movements of the fingers, hand or arm e.g. typists, clerks and routine assemblers.'

On the face of it this should be easier to prove in Court than 'RSI' or non specific pain syndrome. It too however, becomes embroiled in the 'is it organic or psychological' argument and in the absence of identifiable pathological signs it too is difficult to prove in law and few actions are successful.

*Pickford* v. *ICI* (1998) is very instructive in that it demonstrates the views taken by a number of High Court Judges on this condition.

### *(l)* Non Specific Pain Syndrome

This is the most controversial – albeit one of the most common – of all the work related upper limb diagnoses and there are still members of the medical profession who deny its existence. The condition goes under many names including regional pain syndrome, the overuse syndrome, non specific diffuse forearm pain, process worker's arm, occupational overuse injury and, most controversial of all, repetitive strain injury (RSI).

The RSI controversy arises because it contravenes conventional description of a disease process in that there are symptoms but no signs – or at least by the commonly available means of testing for pathological changes. However, as explained elsewhere it remains a very practical term to be used by the general public who known what they mean by it.

The term RSI also implies that an actual 'injury' has been caused by repetitive movements whereas in fact many workers develop their symptoms as a result of static muscle overload rather than dynamic or repetitive movements or the maintenance of constrained posture. Nor is there any pathogenesis which justifies the word 'strain'.

It is a condition diagnosed on exclusion of all the WRULDs here described – and pain referred from elsewhere.

The range of symptoms is so wide and unspecific – pain, aching, tiredness, cramp, weakness, tremor, numbness, swelling, paraesthesia, loss of function – subjective and objective, as to suggest that more than one condition comes under the term non-specific pain syndrome.[39,40]

Chapter 5

# Treatment

*Abstract – Prevention of WRULDs is better than treatment. The aim of treatment is to restore normal function to those tissues which are abnormal. Successful treatment depends on early accurate diagnosis and reflects the severity of the condition. Early diagnosis and treatment can lead to complete recovery but late diagnosis or failure to change working conditions can result in permanent disability. Generally speaking treatment for WRULDs is unsatisfactory.*

Prevention of WRULDs is always better than attempting to cure them and prevention can only be achieved by changes in the working environment. Once a WRULD has been diagnosed then, and with the perfect employer, immediate rest of the affected limb for as long as is required is the best treatment. This perfect state of affairs is, understandably, rarely achieved as often neither employer nor employee can afford such a policy.

The incidence of the WRULD'S – in all their degrees of severity – is much higher than is recorded in the official statistics possibly because so few are recognised for Industrial Diseases Disablement Benefits.[21] Where jobs are difficult to find, and hold, many employees – who under other circumstances would not be prepared to put up with severe musculo-skeletal pain – have no choice but to continue working, live with the problem, and seek ways to ameliorate the pain.[41] This often means using drugs to get through the working day. Masking the natural responses of the body to protect itself however, can in time lead to established, and often irreversible, changes in the soft tissues concerned.

Painkillers and drugs generally have only a limited use in WRULDs, and ice and hot water treatment, physiotherapy, wrist supports, collars and arm straps should be seen as short term measures and not as a means of enabling the patient to continue with unsuitable working conditions.

Successful treatment can only follow accurate diagnosis which is dependent on a comprehensive medical history and physical examination to exclude all other pathological processes. Early reporting of symptoms in the upper limbs is thus essential and preferably should be recorded in the accident book. If the aches and pains can be related to adverse working conditions then simple changes in working procedures, job rotation, better work breaks, ergonomic advice, and sympathetic management may be all that is required.

If this does not solve the problem, or if the soft tissue disorder has progressed to the point where changes in working procedures are insufficient and the symptoms persist, a more positive approach will be required. This usually takes the form of physiotherapy or local steroid injections.

## Physiotherapy

Physiotherapy carried out by those interested and skilled in the specific treatment of WRULDs may be of benefit, particularly in the early stages and before the symptoms persist beyond the working hours. Practical experience however, is that physiotherapy may, at best, be of only short term benefit and, at worst, may stir up the source of the pain and cause the patient even more anguish.

The technique of adverse neural tension has its adherents and many claim to have benefited from it but persevering with long term active exercise regimes and brachial plexus stretching techniques, may do more harm than good particularly if the physiotherapist is inexperienced or when the WRULDs has entered the chronic stage.[42]

An exception to this may be deep massage for tenosynovitis which, if caught early enough, can bring symptomatic relief and permanent changes in signs and symptoms.

## Osteopathy

Many patients gain relief from manipulation of the spine particularly of the cervical spine where degenerative changes are common, and pressure on nerve roots, not uncommon.

The manipulation may have to be repeated quite frequently. Some patients who put the joints of their arms, shoulders and neck through a regular series of gentle loosening up and muscle stretching exercise, even when they are not experiencing upper limb symptoms, seem to benefit.

## Steroid Injections

Cortisone injections, when carried out by an experienced medical practitioner, into the tendon sheath, the pain trigger point joint, carpal tunnel, cervical facets or relevant soft tissue may be curative. More often it gives give some short term pain relief – possibly as much to do with the use of a local anaesthetic with the steroids as anything else – but is an undesirable exercise in the long run and should not be repeated too often. It can also be quite painful. Like many forms of treatment of WRULDs, cortisone is often given on the basis of demand from the patient – 'do something, anything' – and a medical practitioner who is at his wits end having tried everything else will often, understandably, try anything which has not been tried before in the hope of this time striking lucky.

The carpometacarpal joint at the base of the thumb is commonly affected by working activities – before the advent of the washing machine it was described as 'washer woman's thumb'. It is one of the few joints affected by osteoarthritis in which there is a rewarding response to steroid injection – the acromioclavicular joint is another.

**Guanethidine Blocks**

Guanethidine blocks, following an accurate diagnosis of the cause of the pain, can be beneficial.

**Physical Techniques**

The two physical medicine techniques which do appear to offer some relief – particularly in the non specific pain syndrome and tenosynovitis – are the use of the TENS machine and acupuncture.

**TENS**

TENS (Transcutaneous Electrical Nerve Stimulation) is a method of relieving pain by electrical stimulation of nerve fibres via skin electrodes. The author's experience is that many patients benefit from two half hour treatments a day. The TENS machine has the advantage of being under the control of the patient many of whom are able to reduce their intake of pain relieving drugs after a few treatment sessions. TENS machines are not expensive, can often be borrowed from the hospital or GP, are non invasive and non addictive.

**Acupuncture**

It is unclear why acupuncture may benefit the patient – some physicians and surgeons are unenthusiastic about its use – but the author has had some modest success in recommending it.

An electro-acupuncture machine would seem to be more effective than needles. This is essentially a pulse generator, with an altering current transmitted to acupuncture needles via wire leads. The amplitude and frequency of the delivered current can be controlled by the user, as can polarity. Some machines also contain an acupuncture point detector. Most machines run on batteries, and good units have a fail-safe device that protects the patient from excessive current.

Acupuncture does have the disadvantage of the need for regular – and possibly expensive – repeated treatments. However, some GPs now offer this treatment as it cuts down on the use of analgesic drugs.

**Obesity**

Obesity is now the most common adverse health factor in the Western world and the effects of excess weight on musculoskeletal conditions should never be overlooked. A patient will often complain about heavy arms and unspecific shoulder aches and pains and seem surprised when they are told their arms are heavy – from fat – which is putting unnecessary strains upon the muscles of the shoulder girdle. Similarly 'swollen' hands and fingers may be so because of local fat deposits not fluid retention.

Excess weight can also lead to low back, hip, knee and ankle joint degeneration with all the added aches and pains which this entails – as well as the increased fatigue of an already fatigued body. The risk of osteoarthritis in the knee increases by 35% for every 5 kilos of weight gained and a recent (1997/98) study by rheumatologists at St. Thomas' and St. Bartholomew's Hospitals shows that six out of ten cases of osteoarthritis in a study of 1,000 women were due to obesity.

The loss of self esteem can also often become a major factor in an overweight person's life.

**Exercise**

Regular exercise is good for the cardio-vascular system and weight reduction, and by raising the circulating endorphins – and thus the spirits – is beneficial both physically and psychologically.

**Dependence**

The debilitating effect of being physically and psychologically dependent on others as a result of being unable to carry out many routine social and domestic activities for one's self should not be underestimated.

Nor should the disadvantages of accepting the 'victim' mentality.

## Pain Clinics

Pain clinics which support cognitively, whilst not curing the problem, do allow patients to come to terms with their chronic disability.

## Surgery

Surgery has limited value in the treatment of WRULD's and inappropriate surgery can have very adverse effects on the patient.

Surgery is at its most effective in the treatment of carpal tunnel syndrome providing that the diagnosis has been made on the basis of a careful history and physical examination, in the presence of paraesthesia, possibly muscle wasting, and median nerve compression confirmed by nerve conduction tests. In these conditions surgery can be rewarding although it must always be stressed that the relief is of sensory pain distal to the carpal tunnel and not pain or discomfort proximal to the carpal tunnel.

A recent, and encouraging, advance on these traditional surgical techniques has been that of endoscopic carpal tunnel repair.

This procedure is performed under local anaesthetic and fortunately there is no sensation in the flexor retinaculum. Once the area is anaesthetised, a cannula is inserted under the retinaculum at the wrist. A fine endoscope is then inserted alongside the cannula. The endoscope has a retractable cutting blade in a groove on one side, which is withdrawn to divide the retinaculum under direct vision. The whole procedure takes only 15 to 20 minutes and it is possible to operate on both hands in the same session. An improvement on conventional techniques.

Unfortunately, at present, there are only two or three centres in the UK offering the procedure, whereas it is available throughout the USA where the cost effective benefits are well understood.

Most patients are suitable, provided they can lie reasonably still for half an hour. Sutures are removed after 10 days and the hand tends to feel normal two or three weeks after surgery, with full function restored at six weeks.

A prospective trial show that there is less post operative pain with endoscopic surgery than with the open operation for median nerve decompression and patients have more rapid return of pinch and grip strength and are back at work sooner. The results are the same in terms of eventual power with only 1% post operative complications compared to 10% for conventional surgery. As with the open operation the hand is never quite as strong as it was before the carpal tunnel syndrome developed because of pre-operative nerve damage and because at operation part of the pulley system at the wrist is divided – young patients or those with a short history may avoid this.

Surgery may also be recommended to release the common extensor tendon and common flexor tendon at the elbow in the presence of the intractable pain of epicondylitis (tennis or golfer's elbow). The result of this surgery – in the experience of the author – is often disappointing although it may be worth trying if all else has failed. There is also little to be gained – and much to be lost – from surgery for tenosynovitis.

In de Quervain's stenosing tenovaginitis a longitudinal incision over the relevant tendon may be of help – but only if injecting steroids between tendon and sheath has failed.

## Extra Corporeal Shock Waves

Another recent and encouraging development has been the

use of extra corporeal shock waves in chronic calcific tendinitis of the shoulder which is a condition where calcium is deposited around the shoulder joint and tendons causing great pain. About 5,000 pulses of sound shatters the calcium deposits allowing the restoration of full shoulder movements.

**Immobilisation**

Plaster of Paris immobilisation of the affected arm – in the belief that this enforced rest will allow the recovery process time to proceed – is, in the experience of the author, rarely rewarded by symptomatic improvement. It can also lead to muscle atrophy which is difficult to reverse.

**Splinting**

Splinting is also used to rest the limb in the belief – or hope – that the problem will go away. It is rarely successful and may make the condition worse. Resting wrist and hand splints can be useful at night and occasionally during the day but should not be seen as a long term solution.

**Drug Therapy**

When considering drug therapy a wide variety of NSAID (Non steroid anti-inflammatory drugs), antidepressants, muscle relaxants, low dose tricyclics, many different types of pain killers, and local skin applicants have been, and no doubt will continue to be given, with mixed, and often disappointing, results.

It has to be admitted that due to the confusion in the nomenclature of the treated conditions, the absence of specific diagnosis, and lack of properly established clinical studies, there is no real understanding of the effects of the different approaches to treatment. Much is anecdotal.

In the experience of the author avoidance of the activity which caused the problem in the first place; a positive attitude to their disability; regular light exercise; resting the affected limb; whole body warmth; salicylates with meals, and alcohol at bedtime can be as good a treatment regime as the more sophisticated modalities. Sympathy also helps – and reassurance from the medical practitioners involved that the patient has a real and recognised problem.

The end of litigation and the patient's need to constantly dwell on their problems – 'too many doctors and lawyers' – is always beneficial.

# Chapter 6

# Aetiology

*Abstract – WRULDs are caused by the overuse or misuse of a soft tissue beyond the acceptable physiological limit for the individual concerned. This abuse brings about symptoms, such as pain and paraesthesia, and changes in the muscles, tendons and synovial sheaths which may manifest themselves as signs of local swelling, heat, crepitus or restricted movement which may be due to biochemical, membrane permeability or neurogenic changes.*

The exact nature of the changes which take place in the overused soft tissues are largely hypothetical. It is possible that the abnormal mechanical forces on the soft tissues could produce alterations in the levels of metabolic substrates such as high energy phosphates and muscle glycogen, or there could be changes in the shape or composition of muscle tissue, or changes in cell membrane permeability leading to a build up of toxins in cells, the catabolic effect in the tissues exceeding the anabolic leading to a net breakdown of tissue. This in turn could lead to changes in neuro-transmissions.[43•44•45]

If the muscle is constantly fatigued without the opportunity to fully recover this could lead to a state of hypersensitisation of pain receptors which could, in turn, explain why, following the exceeding of physiological limits, the WRULD sufferer finds that quite minor stresses to the affected muscle groups brings immediate aching and pain.[46•48]

The pain receptors presumably become programmed to respond to very weak stimuli and are thus being constantly triggered, or are even continuously active, thus establishing a self sustaining pain cycle which leaves the sufferer vulnerable to pain on carrying out minor domestic tasks involving the musculo-skeletal system or, in the worst situation, being in constant pain.[47•49]

Using the large flexor and extensor muscles of the forearm it would be instructive to see what could be learned from non-invasive magnetic resonance studies of the biochemistry of the muscles in their resting and active state. This could perhaps be associated with basic physiological evaluation of muscle motor control and function.

A possible explanation is that static and dynamic muscle loading has a threshold above which there is impairment of blood flow leading to the accumulation and delayed clearance of metabolites, and, thereby to muscle fatigue.

Certainly a large number of work related changes have been documented as either due to mechanical overload of the muscle tissue or due to metabolic overload. It may take over 24 hours to recover from such overload and if sufficient time for recovery is not allowed self destructive effects may occur within the muscles and toxic substances may well accumulate at the free nerve endings as a consequence of leaky muscle membranes. This means that work related intramuscular changes may be transmitted to the central nervous system as pain.[43–49]

The neuro-muscular programmes of control are clearly very complex and it is not difficult to understand how the neuro-muscular circuitry breaks down when the physiological load is exceeded.

An elegant neurogenic hypothesis of WRULDs has been advanced by Quntren and Elvey[50] which attributes the clinical features of WRULD'S to pathological changes in the cervical spine – nerves, nerve root complex and brachial plexus – or subtle forms of nerve entrapment neuropathy in the upper limbs. It could be tempting to bundle the wide spectrum of hand, arm, shoulder and neck symptoms and signs into this one neurogenic basket but, I fear, this would need to exclude much of what is known about working conditions in factory and office.

There is little doubt that some patients do have a neurogenic component to their WRULDs but this would appear to be the result, not cause, of their problems.

Greening and Lynn (1997) have shown that thresholds for vibration were significantly raised in WRULD'S patients (keyboard workers) with the median nerve being more severely affected than the ulnar or radial nerves. This may indicate a minor polyneuropathy as decreased vibration sensitivity can be an early sign of peripheral neuropathy.[22]

Psychological factors both primary – stress in the work place – and secondary – reaction to adverse social and domestic effects which the onset of upper limb problems can bring – are factors in the aetiology of WRULDs. Stress can be a powerful muscle stimulator and if accompanied by sleep disturbance, can reduce an individuals capacity to recover from fatigue, and thus increase their susceptibility to WRULDs.

*Chapter 7*

# Prevention

*Abstract – Prevention is better than cure and is based on an understanding of the nature of working procedures and the elimination or avoidance of those physical or psychological elements known to be involved in the onset of WRULDs.*

Rarely has the old adage 'prevention is better than cure' been more appropriate than when considering WRULDs, for treatment, particularly in chronic cases, is unrewarding. Yet it is usually possible to prevent the onset of the disorders by an understanding of the nature of the working procedures, vigilance, and the application of well understood principles.

For convenience it is appropriate to consider the workforce procedures as either blue or white collared.

The blue collared work force is involved in many different industrial environments and activities: manufacturing, assembly line, food processing, the service industry, and many different aspects of the clothing industry. The white collared worker is usually some form of computer keyboard, cash register or check out operator.

The things they have in common however, are a preponderance of poorly paid women, working long hours, carrying out repetitive activities, often in poorly designed work stations, in a physically and psychologically disagreeable environment, and with the ever present fear of unemployment.

It is quite extraordinary, as we reach the end of the twentieth century and contemplate the amazing scientific and technological advances of the past fifty years, to realise that so many workers are still forced to put up with conditions for much of their working lives which can best be described as Dickensian – especially as so many of the more unpleasant aspects of their working environment could be improved by the application of common sense and tried and tested shop floor procedures.

The TUC in its 'Wage Rage' report in March 1997 stated that one in four workers is paid less than £4 per hour. Thus five million employees are on less than £4 an hour whilst more than a million of them earn below £2.50 per hour. This is, however, the group which has little choice but to accept the low wages and unsafe working conditions – the alternative is often unemployment – and they are also the group most vulnerable to WRULDs.

Amongst those factors which are well documented as contributing to undesirable working conditions are:

Rapid repetitive movements as part of the working procedures.
Bonus and piece rate systems.
Awkward working positions.
Poor workplace, tool and equipment design.
Excessive work rates.
Lack of job variation.
Inadequate rest breaks.
Process lines being speeded up.
Inadequate training.
Poorly maintained equipment.
Overbearing supervision.
Compulsory overtime.
Monitoring of work rates by machine.
Vibration.
Lack of individual control over the work process.
Returning to work from holiday.

Illness or pregnancy.
Changes in the work process (increased work rate, introduction of new equipment, less variety of tasks).
A knock or blow to vulnerable areas e.g. wrist, elbow etc.
Fear of unemployment.

Many of these undesirable factors are capable of being either eliminated from the work place or improved upon by sensible co-operation between employers and Trades Unions and by inviting the opinions of the worker as to how their working environment can be improved. Too often it is the assembly line worker who is excluded from such discussions, and yet who knows better about how to improve poor working conditions than those forced to put up with them?

More rest breaks, rotation of jobs, reduced rates of work, better training, early involvement of ergonomists, the workers having more say in things which effect them, and medical facilities which allows the early diagnosis of WRULDs, are all factors which can help to prevent WRULDs becoming a problem to the blue collared worker.

When considering the prevention of WRULDs in white collared workers, and whilst accepting that cashiers, check-out operators and filing clerks all risk developing WRULDs, it is the rapidly increasing number of keyboard operators who represent the greatest body of workers at risk from WRULDs.

In the days when typewriters prevailed in the office, WRULDs did not represent a hazard. The typist's hands and arms were in constant use in a variety of movements; putting paper into the rollers manually, returning the carriage after every typed line, stopping to correct mistakes – and there was a low limit to how many depressions of the keys even the fastest typist could carry out.

All that changed with the arrival of the VDU and the computer keyboard.

Instead of the variety of typing movements involving many

different muscle groups, the hands are now held rigid in a position of static muscular tension, often for many hours a day, whilst the fingers can carry out 10,000 to 30,000 fine movements an hour – and often at poorly designed work stations.[27]

The human frame was simply not designed for such activities and it is not surprising they provoke a variety of adverse responses in the soft tissues of the hands, arms, shoulders and back. And it is not only the secretaries who are at risk, for WRULDs are now widespread in all areas of the professions, commerce, industry and journalism where the keyboard is rapidly becoming part of everyday life for many who would never previously have dreamed of doing their own typing. Even children are starting to suffer WRULDs from excessive use of computer games.[26]

The onset of the WRULDs can be manifested as pain, tenderness, swelling, crepitus, pins and needles, numbness and generalised muscle weakness and spasm.

Fortunately there are many ways in which the keyboard operator can be protected from the worst aspects of WRULD'S and the following procedures will benefit all who use a keyboard.

**Posture**

- The feet and thighs should be horizontal and the lower legs and torso vertical. The upper arms should hang vertically down and the forearms should be horizontal. The wrists should be straight. It is very important to keep the elbows in at the sides of the body to minimise any bend in the wrist.
- Chairs must be easily adjustable in height with a single lever releasing a spring or a pneumatic device.
- The display screen and the script being keyed should be just below eye level, with a document holder to neither left nor right but between keyboard and screen if possible.

- The keyboard should be detachable from the screen enabling it to be put at lap level.
- The desk must allow separate and easy adjustment of the screen and keyboard heights.
- The keys should have springs stiff enough to resist the relaxed weight of a finger (approximately 100 grams).
- Keys should have a smooth rather than jarring bottom to reduce vibration. Resting the keyboard on a foam rubber pad helps.
- A rest for the wrists may help although it may impair the blood flow in the hands.
- If possible no more than four hours keying should be done each day.
- No more than 10,000 keystrokes an hour.
- Keyboarding should be broken up as much as possible by other work. Where keyboarding cannot be broken up naturally, a ten minute break should be taken in each hour and other work done, prepared in advance, to take advantage of these breaks.
- Keyboarding staff should become adept at the technique of conscious relaxation of the muscles and special exercises can be done before and after long keyboard sessions.
- There has also been some innovative thought put into the design of the keyboard to make them more ergonomically sound. The Standard QWERTY keyboard requires the hands to be held together with the wrists turned outwards. This action causes the shoulders to be slightly raised and is the position which leads to shoulder and neck aches. By dividing the keyboard into two well separated groups the wrists are held straight which reduces one aspect of the danger of keyboard work. It must be appreciated however, that not all typists can get used to this unconventional keyboard layout.

*Chapter 8*

# Ergonomics

*Abstract – Ergonomists are concerned with fitting the worker to the job and the job to the worker. Early involvement of ergonomic consultants in work place design and layout, and in the design of equipment, machinery and tools, would lead to working conditions conforming to well established ergonomic principles and to a reduction in the number of WRULDs.*

The function of the ergonomist is to make the work place more user friendly and it must always be born in mind that an employer has a duty of care to their employees to achieve that objective. It does therefore, make sense both ethically and commercially to involve ergonomists early on in the design or redesign of the work place.[51•52]

All working environments should be reviewed to assess the strain, discomfort and unnecessary risks placed on the workers due to faulty, ill designed or incorrectly placed machinery. This includes the height of the benches, desks, conveyor belts and seating, and the design of all hand held tools. Ergonomists can make recommendations for re-design of work stations, provision of special tools or the modification of existing tools, and the elimination of badly designed and faulty components. In many cases involving work related injuries, a study commenting on the ergonomics issues is relevant . When ergonomic consultants prepare a report on the ergonomics, health and safety aspects of someone's work and working environment, they typically conduct the following activities.

1. Review in detail the documents related to the project and prepare for the site visit and workplace inspection.
2. Meet the client to gain a better understanding of the job, for example, the system of work as advised by the employer, the practice actually followed, the information and training received, the duration and frequency of different tasks, the existence of any overtime or bonus payments, the equipment used, the environmental conditions in which the work took place, etc.
3. Conduct a site visit to inspect the workplace and collect any relevant details such as the dimensions of the workplace/workstation, the weight and other properties of the load, features of the physical workplace and environment.
4. Read and take into account the reports of any medical experts, prepare a report stating their initial findings and giving their professional opinion. This report can compare their findings with any relevant British Standards or Health and Safety Executive guidance. The report can also be used to determine whether any further ergonomics research is required in support of the case.

These activities can take time and be expensive but many employers find them very cost beneficial in the long term.

*Chapter 9*

# Medico-Legal Aspects

*Abstract – Work Related Upper Limb Disorders are an increasingly common component of personal injury litigation. Whereas Defendants previously preferred to settle out of Court this policy is changing and in future Plaintiffs will need to formulate their claims with great care.*

The magnitude of the WRULD problem is illustrated in the Health & Safety Commission (HSC) 1994/95 Annual Report. Referring to the latest *Labour Force Survey*, the Report says:

> 'Musculo-skeletal disorders were by far the commonest group of self-reported work related conditions . . .'

The Survey estimates there were 593,000 cases of work related musculo-skeletal disorders during the year of which around half were back injuries, 110,000 were upper limb disorders and 58,000 were lower limb disorders.

In the Statistical Supplement to the HSE Report reference is made to a family doctor based survey conducted by the HSE. On Carpal Tunnel Syndrome (CTS) it states:

> 'The GPs judged that approximately half the cases of carpal tunnel syndrome which they saw were either caused or exacerbated by the patient's work . . . this

would imply a national incidence of 20,000 work related cases for which medical advice was sought.'

These figures contrast starkly with the number of workers who actually obtained Department of Social Security Industrial Benefit for musculo-skeletal disorders.

| N1.2 | Year | 1990/1991 | 991/1992 | 1992/1993 | 1993/1994 |
|---|---|---|---|---|---|
| A8 | Tenosynovitis | 556 | 649 | 911 | 800 |
| A4 | Cramp of the hand and foreharm | 46 | 52 | 116 | 135 |
| A5 & A6 | Beat conditions | 187 | 317 | 256 | 257 |
| A12 | Carpal Tunnel Syndrome (prescribed from 1993) | – | – | 20 | 267 |
| A11 | Vibration White Finger | – | – | – | – |
| | **Totals** | **789** | **1,018** | **1,303** | **1,459** |

If the HSC estimates are correct, only 1.3 per cent (13 in every thousand) of those workers who develop a WRULD are obtaining Industrial Injuries Benefit. And these figures do not include the even larger number of patients complaining of upper limb disorders which do not come into the category of prescribed industrial injury.

Almost exactly the same percentage of the 20,000 patients identified by their family doctors as having carpal tunnel syndrome were able to obtain Industrial Injuries Benefit (267) in 1993/94, the first full year that carpal tunnel syndrome was established as prescribed industrial injury. Even allowing for the extraordinary DSS rule that a worker has to be 14 per cent disabled, and the very narrow definition of WRULDs used by the DSS – and which should be expanded – the number managing to receive benefits is very low. Nor is this number in keeping with the DSS's own statistics which show that sickness absence as a result of certain WRULDs increased by 58 percent between 1988 and 1991 – and continues to rise – leading to an annual loss of over 250,000 work days.

## CLAIMING COMPENSATION

Under certain conditions WRULDs are acceptable as an industrial injury in the same way as is noise induced hearing loss, vibration white finger, or the pneumoconioses.

Legal action can be taken against an employer to obtain compensation for industrial injury or disease in the same way as litigation can be initiated for industrial accidents. But compensation is not automatic and the person making the claim must be prepared to prove, in Court, on the balance of probabilities, that the employer had known of the risk to the employee.

In all personal injury actions it is not the employer but their insurance company who defends the action. The TUC's Survey of Union Legal Services suggests that Unions are winning in excess of £5 million a year for WRULD sufferers, a figure which would be enormously increased if all those professionally diagnosed as suffering from WRULDs were compensated. The attitude of insurance companies is however, hardening – and is likely to harden further – and they are increasingly defending WRULD actions, refusing to settle out of Court, and forcing a trial.

Because of this the burden of proof is on the individual to show:

1. He/she has an injury.
2. The injury is work related.

3. The employer should have known of the risk. (Foreseeability)
4. The employer should have taken reasonable care to enable the employee to avoid the risk of injury: but did not do so.
5. He/she must show they have taken reasonable care of themselves and reported to the employer the early onset of their signs and symptoms.

**Items 1 & 2**

These will largely depend on the medical experts witnesses' reports and the expert will, in return, be guided not only by his own medical history and physical examination but also by the GP and hospital records.

**Item 3**

The best way to show 'foreseeability' is to be able to give evidence of what was actually going on in the workplace. To achieve this there are three crucial areas of evidence. Accident book entries: Complaints to management or the company nurse/doctor of symptoms. Union activity: Giving evidence of other workers with similar problems.

*Accident Book* Individuals should be encouraged to make sure that WRULD symptoms are properly entered in the accident book. Records are crucial in any aspect of medico-legal actions and complaints of upper limb problems recorded over a period of months, or even years, will carry great weight in civil proceedings against the employer.

*Complaints of Symptoms* Individuals should be encouraged to report their symptoms to the management and/or the company nurse/doctor as soon as is reasonably possible. This too will result in a written account of the signs and symptoms which will be available for any future litigation.

If a member has been told by their doctor – GP or company

– that he/she has a WRULD but does not inform the employer of this fact, then it will be difficult to blame the employer if the problem gets worse.

*Union Activity* By consulting their members about work place hazards, and inspecting the workplace for risk factors, the Unions representatives may be able to identify possible problems and put the company on notice to set up safety committees with employers, employees and Union representatives.

If the Union representatives follow the systematic approach recommended and put their complaints in writing to the company, keeping copies of any documents, this will be important evidence which can be used in litigation.

Where there is a Union structure and health and safety issue about WRULDs have not been raised – or if raised have not been followed through – the employer's insurers may use this as evidence that there was no real hazard in the work place.

**Item 4**

Showing that the employer has failed to take reasonable care of the employee will take into account the following:

*Basic Systems* The employer should assess the work and monitor the employees for symptoms and, with the use of expert advice and Union consultation, take all practical steps to minimise the risk.

*Warnings* It is impossible to predict who is, and who is not, going to develop a WRULD as different people respond differently to the same working conditions. Thus the employer should regularly warn the whole workforce of any risk and if he fails to do so, knowing there is a risk, this may be held to be negligent.

There are two types of warning:

*Warning at the Start of a Job – Choice* The purpose of this warning is to tell new workers of the risk of the job so that they can decide for themselves whether or not to take it, or to minimise the risks involved in the workplace.

The employer is under a duty of care to provide a safe system of work. If however, a warning has been given and the individual takes the job knowing of the risk then a Court may say that they have accepted the risk and the employer may not be blamed if the employee later develops a WRULD.

If no warning is given and yet the employer knows of the risk then a Court may say that the employer failed to give the employees a proper choice and is responsible for the onset of the WRULD.

It is sometimes construed that if an employee would have taken the job, even if a warning had been given, then the lack of a warning will have made no difference and the employer may not be criticised for that failure alone.

*Warning to Report Systems – Notice* If an employee has been warned that the job carried a WRULD risk and has been told what the dangers are, they are on notice to look out for symptoms and to take steps to protect themselves if they do occur.

If an employee has not been warned and works in ignorance of the risk they may not recognise the symptoms of WRULDs and may make their conditions worse by carrying on working. In this case the employer could be blamed.

If an employee has been warned to report symptoms but fails to do so, then the employer may not be blamed if the condition gets worse, as the Court may consider that the employees have failed to take proper care of themselves.

If employees are warned and they do take steps after the onset of symptoms to report it to the employer and the employer reacts in a way which does not solve the problem or makes it worse – then the employer may be liable.

**Item 5**

Showing the employees have taken reasonable care of themselves.

The Court may blame employees if it considers that they have failed to heed the advice which has been given to them. If an individual has been advised by a medical practitioner to give up the job – and yet carries on working – the Court may say that they have only themselves to blame if the condition gets worse.

No amount of money can compensate an individual who ends up with a serious WRULD problem. If the medical advice is that they are putting themselves at risk by staying in a particular job – and the employer will not take the necessary steps to make the job safer or move the member to a safer job – then the employee should follow medical advice and, if necessary, give up the job. The Court may take the view that people must take responsibility for themselves.

However, it is often a difficult decision to make if there are few other jobs available – the fear of unemployment forces many workers to take risks with their health. This is yet another reason why a good security of employment agreement is essential to protect the interests of individuals who do develop WRULDs.

## Compensation

The amount of compensation will depend on the medical expert's report, the degree of disability, and how permanent any disability is likely to be. Loss of wages and loss of future earnings will also be a factor as will disadvantage on the open labour market.

Compensation may be reduced if the Courts consider there is an element of contributory negligence in that the individual is partly to blame because they failed to look after themselves.

There have been some financially significant awards for WRULDs but generally speaking the Courts have not been generous. It is a sad fact that compensation for pain and sickness is generally low, whilst measurable considerations, such as loss of earnings, rank higher – which is yet another reason why it is important to prevent the onset of WRULDs.

The following factors may also be taken into consideration when preparing an action for WRULDs.

- Details of other employees reporting symptoms even if they do not make a claim.
- Details of Union complaints and activity including copies of relevant documentation.
- Details of all accident book entries applicable to WRULDs and not only to the specific action under consideration but as evidence that others have suffered.
- Details of the pay and productivity systems.
- Details of the systems of work.
- Details of the warnings given at induction and/or otherwise.
- Details of any action the company has taken or failed to take to protect the employee.
- Details of how people with WRULDs are treated including sick leave, transfers, alternative work, job rotation and medical care.

## How to Claim

If an individual believes they are entitled to claim for a WRULD, they should obtain Form Bl 100(b) from their local Department of Social Security (DSS) Office.

The DSS will then arrange a medical practitioner to examine them. The doctor will decide whether or not the employee has an injury which fits one of the prescribed industrial diseases categories and, if so, will assess the degree of disability. Therefore, it is the medical practitioner who will decide whether the individual is entitled to benefit.

The individual will not be entitled to payment of benefit if the doctor decides that their injury does not fit one of the prescribed categories. Even where the doctor agrees that they do have a prescribed disease they will only get benefit if their disablement is assessed at 14% or higher, Many WRULD patients are given assessment below 14%.

If the individual believes they have been wrongly assessed their Union's Legal Department, a welfare rights group, or a private solicitor, can look at their claim and, if necessary, represent them at an Appeal Tribunal.

One of the biggest problems faced by WRULD sufferers when they try to claim Disablement Benefit is that the list of prescribed industrial disease excludes certain types of WRULDs. At present if the person is unfortunate enough to develop 'tennis elbow' or tendinitis in the shoulder, for example, rather than tenosynovitis in the wrist, they will not be entitled to Disablement Benefit because their injury is not included in the prescribed list. Or a patient with diagnosed carpal tunnel syndrome will only receive compensation if the carpal tunnel syndrome is as a result of exposure to vibrating tools and not other occupational activities.

Thus many people who develop WRULDs are, at present, excluded from Disablement Benefit under the rules as they stand.

## Claiming State Benefit

Individuals who develop certain types of WRULDs may be entitled to claim a State Disablement Benefit.

To claim Disablement Benefit the employee must be able to prove:

- They have a prescribed industrial disease.
- It must have developed after 4th July 1948.
- The individual must be in an occupation prescribed for that disease.
- The disease must be caused by that occupation.

As can be clearly seen the government have narrowed the categories of those who can claim by stating that not only must the disease be a 'prescribed industrial disease', the employee must also work in a 'prescribed occupation'.

The prescribed disease categories which concern WRULDs in April 1997 were listed in Leaflet N12 (April 1997) 'Industrial Injuries Disablement Benefit' A4, A5, A6, A7, A8, A11, A12.

Some Unions believe – as does the author of this book – that the present system is unjust and that the list of WRULDs recognised as Prescribed Industrial Diseases should be extended.

However, if an individual is unsuccessful in their claim for Disablement Benefit, because their WRULD does not fit into one of the prescribed categories, it may still be possible to pursue a civil claim for damages against their employer.

## Dismissal On Ground's of Ill Health

Employers should:

- Obtain a proper medical report diagnosing the condition.
- Give the employee the opportunity to comment on that medical report.
- At all times follow their own internal procedures for dismissal.

The question to be answered in all cases is: 'Whether in all the circumstances an employer can be expected to wait any longer for the return to work of an employee and if so, how much longer?'

Employers should also attempt to find alternative work for the employee, rather than resort to dismissal.

It is possible that the Disability Discrimination Act 1995 could affect an employee's rights on dismissal when suffering from a WRULD. Employers are required under this Act to consider reasonable adjustments to the physical workplace, or work station or working arrangements, where an employee can be defined as disabled, which in the terms of the Act means:

> 'A physical . . . impairment which has a substantial and long term adverse effect on ability to carry out normal day today activities.'

The fact that an employee is dismissed 'fairly' for being unfit to do the job for which they were employed does not mean that an employer cannot be sued for common law compensation. Ill health is not an escape route for employers who have a liability to compensate an employee.

The whole area of disability payments was reviewed in 1998 as part of the government's new approach to the Welfare State.

**Civil Compensation**

Compensation from the courts for many injuries including WRULDs is often very low, partly because DSS benefits have to be repaid out of the damages.

As has been explained, employees have to prove that their employer is negligent; that is, the employer failed to take reasonable care for the employee's safety, that the employee was exposed to a reasonably foreseeable risk of injury, and that the fault on the part of the employer led to the condition about which the employee complains.

There are two areas of claim for compensation within a Civil action: Pain and Suffering, and Special Damages.

Compensation for pain, suffering and loss of amenity (the inability to do things they could do before the onset of the condition) is known as General Damages. The level of General Damages is assessed by the Judge depending upon the facts of the case, the medical evidence, and by referring to awards made by other courts for similar injuries in the past. Compensation for General Damages can vary between a few hundred and many thousands of pounds. Each case will be judged on its merits but the medical evidence will often be decisive.

Compensation for financial losses and expenses is known as

Special Damages. This is awarded for those losses and expenses which a Judge accepts arose as a result of a work related condition. Compensation for Special Damages may be awarded for a few weeks, a few months, and in some cases for many years. The claim may be for small amounts such as for painkillers or prescription drugs, or for large sums if a Judge accepts that the condition has led to long term wage loss. Again, every case turns on its own facts but generally speaking it is easier for a lawyer to evaluate financial loss than pain and suffering.

**DSS Benefit Repayment**

Since 1989 the government has required that DSS benefits received by an injury victim should be repaid in full under Special Damages. No repayment is made against General Damages.

The Unions have opposed this unfair law at every opportunity and continues to fight for it to be changed. This situation was however, eased in 1997.

**Three Year Limitation**

The law in the United Kingdom specifies that a claim for personal injury must be brought within three years of the date of the accident, or within three years of an individual believing that their condition was work related.

The Law of Limitation, as this is known, is very strictly applied by the courts. If a WRULD sufferer is in any doubt about whether they have a claim they should initiate proceedings without delay. If a claim is not made within three years of their first realising their condition was work related they may have no claim at all and at best will have to seek leave of the Court for the Court to exercise its discretion to extend the limitation period. For obvious reasons the employer's lawyers will strongly oppose that application.

It may be of value to see laid out the approach which a

barrister will take when giving Advice on Merits when a claim is supported on legal aid:

1. Only if there are reasonable prospects of success can any claim (proposed or otherwise) continue to be supported by a Legal Aid certificate;
2. It is the continuing duty upon those advising a litigant (supported by a Legal Aid certificate) to advise in turn the Legal Aid Board should there be no reasonable prospects of success.
3. Reasonable prospects of success are best defined as a 'better then evens' chance of the recovery of substantial damages (more than nominal) at any anticipated trial.
4. The following elements are required to prove liability:
   (a) *The duty*
   The existence of a foreseeable risk of injury of the kind alleged to have been incurred: the Plaintiff must prove that his/her work was sufficiently intensive to give rise to a foreseeable risk of incurring an injury of the kind which he/she alleges to have incurred, specifically tenosynovitis and more generally a work related upper limb condition ('WRULD').
   (b) *Breach of duty*
   The failure by the Defendant to take steps to extinguish minimise that risk by alteration of work pattern/equipment/training/posture. This would include a failure to provide a safe working environment, i.e. That there were causative ergonomic deficiencies which required remedy.
   (c) *Causation*
   That the pleaded breaches caused the injury complained of. This is an area of great debate in claims of this kind involving work related upper limb disorders (WRULDs).

**Current Situation In Law**

The recent case of *Mughal* v. *Reuters*, *Montenay* v. *Bernard Matthews* and *Moran* v. *South Glamorgan Echo* (High Court in

Cardiff) 11.94 established (and reconfirm) the following:

1. Unless the Plaintiff can show a condition with known pathology the mere fact that he or she suffers pain as a result of performing an activity in the course of employment does not permit recovery: actual injury must be shown as recognised by a body of medical opinion.
2. Both diffuse RSI (in its discreet sense) or a generalised pain syndrome has not been recognised as compensatable injury.
3. No claim alleging RSI or WRULDs simpliciter has succeeded and few are currently being contested. (But see *JL Alexander* v. *Midland Bank*).
4. The futherest that a Judge would currently go to assist a Plaintiff is the following: just as there are those whose susceptibility leads to a specific condition where most would not do so there are those whose susceptibility to pain is such that that which is transmitted along their nerves is indeed greater than most might be expected to experiënce. (See Montenay)
5. A Plaintiff need only show that the negligent work method/process materially contributed to the symptoms giving rise to the injury. Thus even if the injury is constitutional in origin the symptoms may be triggered/accelerated/ brought to light by the work process.
6. Where a Plaintiff's injury is attributable to a number of possible causes, only one of which is the Defendant's negligence, the combination of the Defendant's breach of duty and the Plaintiff's injury does not give rise to a presumption that the defendant has caused the injury: the burden remains on the Plaintiff to prove the link between negligence and injury although that link can be inferred by the evidence.
7. The issue rests upon competent medical evidence.

This situation however, may well be influenced in the

future by the action *J L Alexander and Others* v. *Midland Bank PLC* (22nd May 1998) where his Honour Judge Byrt found for the Plaintiffs – five encoders at Midland Bank.

Judge Byrt held that their condition could either be organic or psychological and in finding for the Plaintiffs stated that although there were no pathological signs – only symptoms – nevertheless their problems were organic.

# Chapter 10

# Health and Safety Executive Regulations

## A Summary of Key Regulations in Relation to Work Related Upper Limb Disorders

*(a) Management of Health and Safety at Work Regulations (1992)*
The Management Regulations oblige all employers to introduce an effective system for protecting the health and safety of their employees. The key points are that employers must:

1. Make an assessment of all the risks to the health and safety of their employees and others who might be affected by work activities.
2. Identify the measures needed to minimise these risks.
3. Make arrangements for the effective planning, organisation, control, monitoring and review of protective and preventative measures.
4. Appoint competent persons to advise on risk assessment and the health and safety measures necessary to eliminate or reduce the risks.
5. Establish clear procedures for dealing with serious and imminent danger.
6. Co-operate and co-ordinate with other employers to ensure that workers are not put at risk by their activities.
7. Provide comprehensive and relevant health and safety information to employees.
8. Provide health and safety training on recruitment or on

being exposed to new or increased risk, in addition to periodic refresher training.
9. Consult in good time with safety representatives whenever there is a potential health and safety problem within their control that could lead to workers being injured.

*(b) The Workplace (Health & Safety) Regulations (1992)*
These Regulations cover all work premises. The Workplace Regulations require employers to ensure that the work environment has:
1. An effective ventilation system, a reasonable temperature and adequate lighting.
2. Sufficient space for employees to work without risk to their health, safety or welfare.
3. Work stations suitable for the people who work there.
4. Adequate and appropriate seating for people at work.
5. Rest areas provided for health and safety reasons.

*(c) The Provisions and Use of Work Equipment Regulations (1992)*
These regulations deal with the correct selection and use (including starting, stopping, operation, maintenance, transport and cleaning) of work machinery, appliances, tools, plant and equipment. The regulations are very wide ranging. For example, machinery could be anything from a dumper truck to a VDU, and tools could include both a shotgun and a stapler.
The regulations require employers to comply with the following general requirements:
1. Ensure that work equipment is suitable for the task for which it is used. Take into account working conditions and hazards when selecting equipment.
2. Ensure that appropriate information, instruction and training is given to employees, supervisors and managers.
3. Ensure that all new equipment complies with relevant legal standards.

Other more specific requirements must also be met. Employers must ensure that work equipment:

1. Is maintained in efficient working order and that dangerous parts are effectively guarded.
2. Has suitable control systems and control devices.
3. Is stable and clamped or otherwise secured where necessary.
4. Is marked and has clear warning devices, where necessary for reasons of health and safety.

Although these Regulations came into effect on lst January 1993, some requirements were phased in and the regulations were fully in effect on lst January 1997. Employers also have to ensure that any equipment purchased meets the requirements of the Machine (Safety) Regulations 1992, which came into effect on lst January 1995.

These three sets of regulations outlined above are general, applying to most workplace health and safety problems. It should however, be fairly

obvious that the conditions which can cause WRULDs are encompassed in these general regulations – management, in other words, have no excuses for not acting to prevent any such injuries.

The following regulations are more specific and are directly related to WRULDs.

*(d) Manual Handling Operations Regulations (1992)*

These regulations are very important. They cover the whole range of manual handling activity involving the transport or support of loads. This includes lifting, lowering, pushing, pulling, carrying or moving any load, by hand or by bodily force. The Regulations are not limited to heavy loads. Loads that are not particularly heavy can pose risk because of their size, the nature of the contents or because they are awkward to handle.

The risk assessment under the Management Regulations

(outlined above) should show whether there is a manual handling risk. If there is, a detailed assessment is then required under Regulation 4 of the Manual Handling Regulations.

The guidance to the Regulations stresses the importance of risk assessments, taking account of:

1. Posture, twisting movements, stooping or reaching upwards.
2. Excessive lifting, lowering, pushing or pulling.
3. Any frequent or prolonged physical effort.
4. Work paced by a machine.

Employers are required to:

1. Arrange work to avoid manual handling where possible (this could mean job redesign or bringing in mechanical lifting aids.)
2. Use the risk assessment to implement preventive and protective measures to reduce the risk or injury to employees from unavoidable manual handling.

   Risk assessments under the Manual Handling Regulations can cover many of the types of jobs that cause WRULDs and employers should use the Manual Handling Regulations to protect their employees who are at risk.

*(e) Health and Safety (Display Screen Equipment Regulations) (1992)*

The Health and Safety (Display Screen Equipment Regulations), established for the first time, minimum health and safety standards for VDU (Visual Display Unit) users. They cover systems of work and the suitability of the equipment and workstation. All equipment that was purchased after 31st December 1992 must meet these minimum legal standards. Older workstations must comply by 31st December 1996, or sooner if a risk assessment has identified problems that need rectifying.

Employers must:

1. Analyse all workstations to assess the risks to the health and safety of display screen equipment users, and reduce the risk identified as far as is reasonably practicable.
2. Plan work activities so that users have periodic breaks or changes of activity from screen use. The GMB recommends a mixture of screen based and non screen based work or if this is not possible a minimum ten minute break every hour.
3. Provide users upon request with an appropriate eyesight test, and special corrective appliances if the test shows these to be necessary. Tests and any spectacles required for screen based work must be paid for by the employer.
4. Provide adequate information to users about all aspects of health and safety relating to their workstations and the measures taken by the employer to comply with the Display Screen Equipment Regulations.

The Display Screen Equipment Regulations and related Guidance provide details about the safety of systems of work and work equipment. This includes the display screen, keyboard, workstation, chair, working environment and the computer software used.

The employer should consult Trade Union Safety Representatives over all of those aspects.

Employers must not use equipment to monitor the performance of workers without their knowledge.

# Chapter 11

# Case Histories

## Carpal Tunnel Syndrome in a Potato Sorter

Mrs Gray's husband is an agricultural worker and they live in a tied cottage. Initially, Mrs Gray did not work but, in January 1992 at the age of 25 she was offered part time work sorting potatoes. There were no problems at first but she gradually increased her hours until she was working full time.

Her hours of work were from 8.30 am to 4.00 pm with a 15 minute break in the morning, half an hour for lunch, and sometimes a 15 minute break in the afternoon. She was working on a primitive conveyor belt, in an open shed in the farm yard, without heating, and during the winter – which was the busy time of the year – the working conditions were at their worst, being both cold and wet. She was also forced to work overtime.

The potatoes arrived from all parts of the world often with soil adhering to them and there was a system of cleaning by which the potatoes were tipped into a hopper and scrubbed by jets of water. They emerged from the bottom of the hopper on to the conveyor belt and it was Mrs Gray's job to discard all those potatoes which failed to conform to one of the four required sizes – small to jumbo – or were green or rotten.

The potatoes came by in front of her at a speed which allowed her to reach forward, grasp one in each hand using fingers and thumb, and then throw the potatoes backwards over her shoulders into a bin.

The potatoes were wet from the hopper and although she wore gloves and was provided, finally, with a protective apron, she was often cold and wet soon after she started work and remained so all day.

The amount of potatoes she dealt with varied throughout the year but during the busy winter months she would sort between 2 and 5 tons of potatoes a day.

Management insisted she needed to identify up to 200 reject potatoes a minute using both hands and if she failed to keep up with the speed of the conveyor belt the potatoes could bulk up further down the line and caused irritation amongst other workers.

There was also much lifting of bags and general labouring activities in and around the potato packing unit. She would have liked to have had changes in her working routines but her requests for a change were ignored and she would thus need to spend seven or eight hours a day mainly sorting the potatoes.

In the summer of 1994, she started to develop paraesthesia in the right (dominant) hand. This took the form of pins and needles in the thumb, first, second, third and forth fingers. She then developed similar symptoms on the left – but she put up with the pain by using paracetamol before she started work and again during the day.

The records show she saw her GP in November 1995 who wrote to a consultant surgeon stating that Mrs Gray had: '*bi-lateral carpal tunnel syndrome – worse on the right*'.

She was seen by an orthopaedic consultant and, following nerve conduction tests, he confirmed the carpal tunnel syndrome. Surgery for decompression of the right median nerve took place in April 1996 and in September 1996 for the left hand.

Surgery was successful but both hands were weaker than before the operations.

Mrs Gray finally found the bad working conditions, poor man-management and the general unpleasantness of the senior staff too much to take and gave up the job.

*Discussion*

It is not apparently in question that Mrs Gray worked as a potato sorter under conditions which could at best be described as primitive. She worked long hours sorting up to five tons of potatoes a day, with few breaks, in cold wet surroundings and for an employer who appeared complacent about the arduous nature of the working environment, disinterested in improving Mrs Gray's conditions and unsympathetic to her medical problems as they gradually emerged.

She asked for her work to be varied and for others to take over some of her less pleasant and more arduous duties but her requests were refused and she finally developed, and needed treatment for, carpal tunnel syndrome.

Although there are other causes of carpal tunnel syndrome than those which are work related none of these causes applied to Mrs Gray and, on the balance of probabilities, it was accepted that her problems were work related.

As however, her husband did not wish to risk losing his job on the farm and their tied cottage it was decided not to pursue an action for personal injury.

## Tenosynovitis in a Chicken Process Worker

Mr Brown started to work at the chicken processing factory in April 1995. At this time the company policy was to rotate the workers around a series of chicken processing areas so as to prevent employees spending long periods carrying out any particular procedure.

The employees thus spent time in the portion hall picking up pieces of chicken and laying them out according to a certain agreed order; in the grading room putting chicken pieces on trays; at the grading belt; hanging up the fresh chickens by the wings on the chill conveyor belt; and in eviscerating chickens, identifying and isolating the livers.

Mr Brown had no problems whilst working in the portion hall, grading room or on the grading belt but found – about two months after starting work – that he was having problems whilst working on the chill conveyor belt.

The chickens moved past him on the conveyor belt having been killed, defeathered, lacking heads and feet, and weighing on average about five pounds. The working procedure involved taking hold of the thighs of a chicken using both hands with fingers flexed around the thighs and the thumb held stiffly so as to press down against the lower part of the leg. The body and neck were directed towards the processor and, by holding the chicken in this position, he was able to lift it and place it into a V-shaped shackle which was moving by at about eye level.

He was expected to hang 35 chickens every minute and if he failed to keep up this pace he was criticised by the team leader as the chickens would then accumulate and cause disruption to the other members of the team.

He had been working at this procedure for about two weeks when at 2.30 pm one day he developed pain in the right wrist in the area of the radial styloid. The pain quickly extended into his fourth and fifth fingers and he could feel his fingers starting to swell within his glove. He went to see the first-aider and was given a bandage but told he must return to the conveyor belt. For the next four hours of the shift he continued working using his first, second and third fingers and thumbs whilst trying to protect fingers four and five. Although in great pain he finished the shift and recalls that his complaint was put into the accident book. (Unfortunately this book is stated to have been later lost in a fire so was not available). The next day his hand was still bandaged, swollen and painful but he started as usual at 6.00 am and worked until noon – still unable to use his forth and fifth fingers.

The following day he was moved on to the processing of chicken livers. This involved thrusting his hand into the chicken's abdominal cavity via the cloaca, grasping the gullet and, with a twisting and pulling movement, removing the entire abdominal contents. It was then his duty to identify the liver and place it on a separate tray – the remaining viscera being used elsewhere. The evisceration manoeuvre involved flexing the fingers tightly around the gullet with the right thumb pressed down hard across fingers one, two and three. This position protected fingers four and five and he was able to continue throughout the working day.

The following day he telephoned the company to say that his fingers were swollen and he was in such pain that he was unable to carry on work. He went to see his GP who referred him to the local hospital where he was given splints and pain killers which allowed him to return to work on the chill conveyor belt the following day. However, the pain again returned and he describes how, although he wore gloves, he was constantly knocking and grazing his hand as well as suffering from what the general practitioner had by then described as tenosynovitis.

He continued working and visiting his GP but the condition failed to improve and in September 1995 in an effort to keep his wrist immobile the hospital put his right arm in a plaster of Paris cast from the elbow to the mid hand. At the end of three weeks the plaster cast was removed but he had no significant benefit from this treatment for, as soon as he returned to work, the hand swelled up.

He was then signed off for three months over the Autumn/Christmas period. In January 1996 he saw the company doctor who told him that he should be taken off the chilled hanging and liver evisceration areas. This advice was not implemented by management and he returned to work as usual after a short period of lining trays – an activity which he could do without too much of a problem especially as he was taking pain killers during the day.

At this time, because of the continuing pain and the discomfort, he was inevitably favouring the right hand and arm and making more use of the left. In particular he changed over to using his left hand when he was eviscerating the chickens. This meant that when he thrust his hand into the abdominal cavity he was rotating his left hand in a supination/pronation movement to the left, flexing all the fingers with the thumb pressed across the first and second fingers. This was an uncomfortable movement and he quickly developed pain at the base of the left thumb and forefinger. As the eviscerating manoeuvre also involved pulling he needed to involve the flexor muscles of the elbow and wrist and, as a result, he developed an area of acute pain on the flexor aspect of the left forearm.

Thus at this stage he was suffering pain in the thumb, first, second and third fingers and forearm on the left, and pain and swelling in the fingers of the forth and fifth fingers on the right.

He visited his GP again who laid him off work and referred him to the hospital for physiotherapy which was of no benefit.

As it was apparent he could not carry out his duties he was sacked from the chicken processing factory in September 1996 and he has not been able to return to work since.

As a result of these problems he has constant aching and pains in both hands. Many of the mundane, social and domestic activities are beyond him. His girlfriend has to prepare his food as he finds even buttering a piece of bread is often too painful a procedure for him to carry out.

His girlfriend also does most of his shopping for if he goes himself he has to carry the shopping in shifts as there is a low limit to how much weight his hands can take. He cannot shave because of the difficulties in holding a razor and has had to grow a beard. He also finds washing difficult and has been forced to limit himself to showering. He cannot lie easily in one position and, in particular, when he is watching television he has to constantly move the position of his hands to prevent the development of pins and needles – particularly over the forth and fifth fingers.

*On Examination*

The tendons of the left abductor pollicis longus, extensor pollicis brevis and extensor pollicis longus muscles were prominent and appear to be tender on palpation – particularly extensor pollicis brevis.

The left hand is also exquisitely tender on palpation at the base of the left thumb and on movements of the fingers – particularly movements involving extensor indicis and extensor carpi radialis brevis. Other movements of the wrist were also painful.

On the right there is no tendonitis but he indicates limitation of movement with pain in fingers four and five, and points to an area across the back of the hand which is painful on flexion and extension of all fingers. Pain is also present on palpation over the ulnar styloid and the inner aspect of the wrist.

*Discussion*[53]

It does not appear to be in question that Mr Brown suffered pain and discomfort – first in his right hand and then in his left hand – as a result of the repetitive movements involved in the preparation of chicken carcasses. His GP made a diagnosis of tenosynovitis and the doctors at the local hospital largely agreed with this diagnosis.

When examined a year after the events the inflammatory changes were still present on the left along the course of the tendons of the main extensor muscles to the thumb – abductor pollicis longus, extensors pollicis longus and brevis.

These three are the main muscles involved in extension movements of the thumb – that is the movements involved with hanging chickens by their legs and eviscerating carcasses.

*Opinion*

The medical opinions were that Mr Brown was suffering from tenosynovitis of the tendons of abductor pollicis longus, and extensor pollicis longus and brevis on the left, and the medical records demonstrate he has previously suffered tenosynovitis in the right hand and wrist.

This condition is work related and, on the balance of probabilities, arises out of the repetitive nature of his work at the chicken processing plant.

The action is ongoing.

## Non Specific Pain Syndrome from Excessive Keyboard Work

Mrs Green was first employed by an electric wholesalers in November 1985 and she had no significant problems with her hands or arms until the annual stocktaking in June 1994.

At the time in question she was aged 34 and had already worked a normal week when she was requested by management to carry out an urgent stocktaking over the weekend of the 17th, 18th and 19th June. She had the task of keying in to the computer database the stock records compiled by about six men. This information was delivered to her as stocktaking sheets of paper containing five digit part numbers, three digit colour codes and two digit location codes of may thousands of items of electrical goods held in stock. It was arduous, detailed work which she carried out in working conditions which, from her description, were ergonomically poorly designed. She did however, finish the stocktaking only to be told on the Monday morning that some of the information provided to her had been falsified and the whole exercise would need to be repeated the following weekend. She therefore, worked a normal full week and again over the 24th, 25th and 26th June she completed the painstaking exercise of the stocktaking. She was then informed on the Monday that again there had been errors in the stocktaking and that the entire procedure would need to be repeated for a third time.

She completed the stocktaking for a third time but at this point she started to get pain, aching and swelling in her wrists. In spite of these problems she persevered at work for a further month and then saw her general practitioner who diagnosed tennis elbow, gave her some anti-inflammatory drugs and laid her off work. However, the condition did not improve with rest and over the following year it gradually worsened to the point where her right hand was too painful for her to use the mouse and she thus started to key in the information using the left hand. Unfortunately by favouring the right hand in this way she placed too much of a burden on her left hand which also started to give her trouble.

As a result of this she was finally incapable of carrying out any computer work, was laid off in October 1995, made redundant in January 1996 and she has not been able to work since.

She was seen by a consultant physician with an interest in work related upper limb disorders, who diagnosed 'repetitive strain injury' in October 1995. She has had regular physiotherapy sessions since January 1995 and has been treated with three steroid injections into the shoulders.

When seen in 1997 there had been some improvement over the previous eighteen months. The hands did not swell as they did previously, although she still finds it difficult to wear her rings, doesn't like having her hand held, needs to support the right hand on a pillow when sitting in a car – and turning knobs, opening tins and bottles and carrying anything of any weight all caused pain. Gardening and housework is now largely under the control of her husband and dress making, which she previously greatly enjoyed, is no longer possible as she cannot hold or thread a needle. Thus many of the routine domestic and social activities are either difficult or impossible for her to carry out.

On examination, power was reduced in both hands but more so on the right, although there was no loss of muscle bulk, she was able to flex and extend at the wrists and supinate and pronate but these movements were carried out slowly and painfully; she indicated pain over the base of the fingers two, three and four; the back of the hand, and along the extensor muscles; she was tender to pressure over the flexor retinaculum and her fingers were cold.

*Discussion*

In many ways Mrs Green is classical of the type of person who develops a work related upper limb disorder. These sufferers are typically the most hard working, conscientious female employees: women who are always willing to respond to a challenge, work overtime, stand in for absent colleagues, and they are known by their employers to be the employee who will best respond to an emergency situation.

When Mrs Green refers to herself as 'a perfectionist' she probably summarises the characteristic of many of those women who develop the overuse syndrome – for this is not a syndrome which occurs among those who are irresponsible or idle. It is a risk only to those who can pull out all the stops when requested to do so.

There can however, be a price to be paid for this conscientiousness and this comes when the only-too-willing employee responds to a challenge, as did Mrs Green, but then exceeds the physiological limits of their soft tissues.

This was the situation faced by Mrs Green in June 1994. To complete a complicated and detailed data entry exercise in the first place – when many others would have refused to work over a weekend – and then to need to repeat the procedure not twice but three times was an exercise far beyond the call of duty.

Until that time Mrs Green had had no problems with her hands and arms and there can be little doubt that the sudden development of pain in her hand was related to the excessive demands made upon her soft tissues by the intense keyboard work over those three weekends in June 1994.

She was also typical in that, although she had the classical symptoms of a WRULD, she had no signs of pathology which could be measured or assessed.

The medical opinion however, was that on the balance of probabilities the intensity of the keyboard work and the stresses which this induced in June 1994 caused a work related upper limb disorder which manifested itself as a non specific pain syndrome.

The action was settled out of Court.

## Non Specific Regional Pain Syndrome in a Computer Operator

Mrs Smith, a 45 year old legal secretary had worked for a firm of solicitors for about 10 years without any medical problems until there was a sudden change in the nature and pressure of her work.

Her usual hours of work were Monday to Friday 9.00 am to 5.00 pm – although she would invariably work an additional hour each evening to enable her to finish that day's work. However, the usual hours were a rarity as the firm was very busy and she was happy to earn the high salary which came with overtime.

Her work was essentially that of a computer operator with very little real secretarial work involved. She was at her computer for anything up to fifteen hours a day, when working overtime, with 12 hours a day at the VDU being common place. There were no official breaks in the morning or afternoon and although she took twenty minutes at lunch time and occasionally twenty minutes at 9.00 pm before the canteen closed, she was essentially spending her entire working day, and much of the night, typing. Even in the less busy period she would normally not get home before midnight.

The firm of solicitors was open for business 24 hours a day and in the autumn of 1995 during a particularly busy four month period Mrs Smith worked from 9.00 am to 3.00 am the following morning – six days a week.

She was apparently a highly competent word processor operator and she describes how her fingers were faster than the computer and at times she had to stop in order for the computer to catch up.

She started to develop pains in the hands in late 1995, initially in her left hand but then in her right, and finally involving her elbows. At times the pain would extend up to the shoulders.

At first the pain would come on late in the working day and disappear if she were able to return home and relax in the evening. Later however, the pains started to appear earlier in the day until, finally, they were present throughout the working day, during the evening, and kept her awake at night.

She took paracetamol to mask the pain and allow her to get through the working day and when she saw the company doctor she, whilst being unhappy at the intensity of Mrs Smith's work, suggested some stronger form of pain killer should be used to allow her to continue to carry out her duties.

She saw her GP in December 1995 and was given an anti-inflammatory drug which was of no benefit to her. In June 1996 she was referred to a consultant rheumatologist who carried out a spectrum of pathology tests, all of which were normal.

By August 1996 the problems in Mrs Smith's hands were

worse and the rheumatologist suspected '*it could be the overuse syndrome*' and organised nerve conduction studies and isotope bone scans of her hands – all of which were normal. He also provided her with resting splints to use in bed at night. By October 1996 carpal tunnel syndrome was mooted and she had nerve conduction tests and injections into the left carpal tunnel – without benefit – nor was physiotherapy and acupuncture.

Her employers put her on light duties for a few months and she saw a number of other doctors and had other treatments – none of which helped. Her employment was terminated in August 1997 as she was unable to carry out her keyboard duties.

When seen by the author in Spring 1998 she had been unable to carry out any keyboard work for over a year and there was constant, underlying aching in her hands and fore-arms, associated with pins and needles.

Although she has learnt to live with these problems many of the routine household, social and domestic activities are achieved only with pain or by pacing herself to avoid doing too much at one time. To reduce her workload she has had to buy a dishwasher, use a new type of hoover, but she is unable to garden or drive her car and even the simplest things like holding up a newspaper can be beyond her.

Her hands and arms showed loss of muscle bulk over the thenar eminence particularly on the right, her grip power was reduced, there were changes in sensitivity over her finger tips, and pronation and supination were painful. She indicated the pain as passing from the wrist to just below the elbows.

*Discussion*

It is not in doubt that Mrs Smith worked extraordinary long hours under conditions which are surprising in this day and age. At times she was working from 9.00 am to 3.00 am the following day with very few breaks and under conditions which must have been very tasking to her musculo-skeletal system in the back, shoulders, arms and hands. Much of the time was spent typing and she would work fairly continuously for 12 to 15 hours a day, six days a week. Not surprisingly, her soft tissues rebelled at such physical abuse and she developed various aches and pains in her arms and hands which were variously described by the rheumatologist as 'carpal tunnel syndrome', 'overuse syndrome', 'regional pain disorder' or 'RSI'.

What all these terms amount to is that the intensity of the keyboard work caused her to exceed the physiological limits of her soft tissues and she developed a work related upper limb disorder best described as a non specific regional pain syndrome which led to her being unable to continue with her well paid work.

The action is ongoing.

## Epicondylitis in a Machinist

Mrs Jones was employed as a machinist in a foundry between 1972 and 1994, mainly hand-finishing a variety of metal components made from cast iron and brass. She was on bonus work and was provided by her employers with a list of the number of the different components she was expected to finish in an hour and, if she failed to achieve that output, she was not allowed access to the higher piece rates.

In the case of door locks she was expected to clean off, using a firm grinding wheel, a basic three hundred items per hour but would often achieve an output of three hundred and fifty an hour – representing up to four thousand items during the working day.

The cast iron door locks were delivered to her work station in the rough case form by a labourer and she needed to bend over using both hands to pick up a door lock from the container. She then held the lock against a rotating grinding wheel moving it around in her hands so as to clean off the surfaces where they were rough from the die casting. These manoeuvres involved holding her arms out from the shoulder and bent at the elbows so as to forcibly bring up the casting against the rotating wheel. She was provided with gloves and a visor to protect her face from the metal dust. Force was necessary as holding the lock loosely could allow it to be thrown out of her hands.

Thus for the duration of her 12 hour working day – for she always accepted overtime – she was standing with her arms in a semi flexed position at the elbows, and extended at the shoulders, with her hands moving in different directions at the wrists – flexion, extension, pronation and supination – as the door lock was manipulated against the rotating wheel.

She started work at 8.00 am, took half an hour unpaid meal break at lunch time, and then worked through to 8.00 pm to gain four hours overtime. She had a half hour paid break at about 6.00 pm and would often work on a Saturday morning.

In about 1992 she started to develop pains in the right shoulder and was given a hydrocortisone injection which helped for a while. By 1993 however, her GP notes record that she was developing pains in the elbows and shoulders

Her pains persisted and her GP, having made a diagnosis of epicondylitis, referred her for specialist opinion and treatment – with little benefit to her.

She was given various types of pain killers by the general practitioner which allowed her to work through the pain. She also complained to the nursing staff at the factory about her elbow and was provided with a spray to numb the pain and given Paracetamol to allow her to continue working. She was also given stronger drugs by her GP but found she was getting dizzy whilst working and discontinued taking them.

So for a period of about six years she was masking the symptoms of epicondylitis by the use of analgesic spray, different types of pain killers, and an arm strap, all of which allowed her to continue whilst the underlying condition was worsening and, ultimately, becoming intractable. She also developed various gastric problems related to the pain killers.

By 1994 the pain in her arms was becoming unbearable and affecting her life outside the factory both day and night and even on holiday. By 1995 she could not continue and her doctors advised she retire on medical grounds. She has not worked since 1995.

She now suffers from chronic pain in the elbows and needs to take eight strong pain relieving tablets a day and more at night to alleviate the symptoms and allow her some sleep. She has been doing this for three years, and for the previous ten years was mainly taking a combination of codeine and Paracetamol until they started to have an effect on her eye sight and gut.

She now has to allow her husband to do many of the routine domestic and social activities around the house – hoovering, preparing the vegetables, carrying the shopping – as the pain and disability in her arms makes many of these routine tasks either extremely painful or impossible to carry out.

She finds it difficult to sleep and has had to come to terms with the fact that the pain and discomfort are to be a permanent part of her life.

On examination in 1997 she was unable to bend down and touch her toes because of the difficulty in fully extending her arms. The inner (medial) aspects of both elbows demonstrates pain on all movements and palpation over the medial epicondyle is exquisitely painful. She was also painful on palpation over the lateral elbow joints and anterior aspect of the forearms and, specifically, the flexor carpi radialis, pronator teres, and the supinator muscles.

*Discussion*

Mrs Jones worked on the foundry assembly line for nearly 30

years carrying out a variety of tasks all of which involved the repetitive movements of her hands and forearms for many thousands of times a day, with few breaks, and under conditions which put profound arduous stresses and strains on her musculature. This work had by 1994 already produced aches and pains in her elbows which needed to be masked by pain-killers to allow her to continue in her work.

She saw a number of specialists and had a variety of treatments none of which were of much benefit to her. This is probably due to the fact that she has developed irreversible soft tissue changes – particularly in the flexor muscles of the forearms – as a result of the many years of arduous work and the use of pain killers.

At various times she was diagnosed as having 'golfer's elbow' or 'tennis elbow' both of which are probably inflammatory conditions at the point of origin of the extensor and flexor muscles respectively.

The pronator teres muscle rotates the radius upon the ulnar turning the palm of the hand backwards i.e. it pronates the forearm and hand. It also helps to flex the elbow joint when great force is required. The pronator muscle prevents separation of the lower range of the radius and ulnar when upward thrusts are transmitted through the carpal bones from the hand. The pain and weakness in these muscles would fit in with the constantly repeated movements of the hands and forearm. As these are the principle activities being carried out by Mrs Jones, it is understandable that these are the muscles which have suffered most from the many years of hard work.

*Prognosis*

It is now three years since Mrs Jones stopped working and there has been little improvement during this period. It is likely she will need to learn to live with her problems for the rest of her life. She is now aged 51.

*Opinion*
Mrs Jones is suffering from a bi-lateral work related upper limb disorder manifesting itself as an epicondylitis involving the forearm flexor muscles, and in particular, the flexor carpi radialis, but also the muscles involved in supination and pronation movements of the hands and wrists, and arising out of the nature of her work in the foundry during the period 1972 to 1995.

A settlement was agreed out of Court.

## Rotator Cuff Syndrome in a Plasterer

Mr John was a 48 year old self employed plasterer. He had originally carried out a five year apprenticeship but when seen had been employed on his own behalf for twenty years.

He was paid on yardage – that is, the builder would subcontract the plaster work to Mr John and his labourer and they would measure the area to be plastered in square yards. A price for the job would be agreed with the builder and Mr John would be paid on completion of the work – whether it took a short time or a long time although in general he was always under pressure to finish the plastering as soon as possible to allow the other trades to carry on with their work.

He would usually start at 7.00 am and, allowing about 20 minutes for the labourer to knock up the first quantity of plaster, would then be working for as many as 12 hours a day, taking breaks as required. This usually meant half hour at lunch time and ten minute breaks in the morning and afternoon but he was always anxious to keep the rhythm of the work going in order to finish the job as soon as possible.

The method of work was for the labourer to mix up the plaster in hundred weight quantities and about 7 lbs at a time would be placed by the labourer on Mr John's plastering board which he held in the left hand by a handle beneath the board.

He carried out the actual plastering by means of a long trowel which he worked with the right hand transferring the plaster from the board to the wall in qualities of about 1 lb at a time.

The work was physically demanding in that he was both supporting the heavy weight in the left hand whilst the right hand, forearm, arm and shoulder were in continuous movement applying and smoothing the plaster throughout the long working day and always concerned that the plaster would dry before it was used.

The work was particularly difficult when the right arm was raised above the head when plastering a ceiling as the arm was held abducted and elevated for long periods which placed a considerable burden on the right shoulder joint and the surrounding muscles and ligaments.

Mr John had various aches and pains over the years in the right shoulder, and to a lesser extent in the left arm from the weight of the plaster, but he had accepted this as part of the expected problems of plastering. It was only when he returned from holiday that the aches and pains in both arms and shoulders were significant and he usually needed to work for about a week before the pains subsided. During this week he would quite often use pain killers to mask the pain and allow him to carry on.

He continued with this type of work until one day whilst he was plastering a ceiling he suddenly developed an acute pain in the right shoulder which was particularly painful over the tip of the shoulder when the arm was abducted – although there was also pain when he rotated his arm as part of the plastering procedure. He tried to protect his arm as best he could but towards the end of the day he found the right shoulder too painful to continue and he went to see his GP.

His GP advised him to take time off work but Mr John was under contract to finish the job and was forced to carry on for a further three days masking the pain in the shoulder with painkillers every three hours.

On examination he was found to be an extremely well built man with the musculature of the chest, back, both arms and shoulders, extremely well developed. He was however, acutely painful on palpation over the supraspinatus muscle on the right and he demonstrated a painful arch on active movements of the right arm in abduction, particularly when he lifted the arm above 80 degrees.

There was pain in the deltoid region and pain particularly on resisted active movements such as those which caused abduction of the supraspinatus, external rotation of the infraspinatus and the teres minor muscles, and on internal rotation of the subscapularis.

*Discussion*

It was clear that Mr John was suffering from rotator cuff tendonitis. He was advised that this condition would become worse if he continued to work as a plasterer as the abnormal movements of the right arm particularly when plastering above the horizontal would lead to further degenerative and inflammatory changes in the right shoulder.

He tried, but he was unable to continue working, and was finally forced to allow his son to do the plastering whilst he carried out the duties of the labourer.

## Sheath infections of the Hands in a Tradesman

Mr Evans was a 54 year old industrial electrician. He was the maintenance electrician in a factory mainly dealing with the electrical systems controlling conveyor belts.

On the day in question he was using a screw driver to replace a fuse box in an awkward position beneath one of the conveyor belt supports. The screwdriver slipped and penetrated the palm of his right hand.

He was not particularly concerned about the injury and

merely washed his hands and applied a local plaster. He then returned to his normal duties. He did not report the accident to the first-aider on duty and it was not recorded in the accident book.

Later that day however, he developed a throbbing pain in the palm of the hand and, although this was uncomfortable during the night, he was able to report for duty the next morning. The pain had now become worse and he had difficulty in holding his screwdriver so he went to the first-aider who advised him he had a local infection, swabbed the wound with antiseptic, gave him a plaster and he returned to work.

The pain persisted, there was some local swelling, but in spite of the pain he worked for the rest of the day and went to see his GP in the evening. By this time the pain was severe, throbbing and there was intense local tenderness and some loss of function of the hand.

His GP referred him to the local hospital casualty department and he was seen by the doctor on duty who diagnosed a pulp infection of the hand, gave him antibiotics and suggested he return the next day.

When he did return to the hand clinic he was running a temperature, the hand was intensely painful and the pain and swelling had extended from the palm of the hand to the wrist on the flexor surface, and all movements of the hand were intensely painful.

The orthopaedic surgeons diagnosed septicaemia of the ulnar bursae which had now extended to behind the flexor retinaculum and surgery was required.

He was given a general anaesthetic, an incision was made over the ulnar bursa and he was given intravenous antibiotics. He remained in hospital for three days with the hand suspended to encouraged drainage.

He made a reasonable recovery but needed to have antibiotics and painkillers for the next two weeks and was, in all, three weeks off work.

## De Quervain's Stenosing Tenovaginitis in a Textile Worker

Mrs Pitt was a 37 year old textile worker who, except for an eight year gap during which she had her children, had worked in the same mill since she left school. The nature of her work had changed over the years but when seen in December 1996 she had been working at the same specific job in the mill for the previous seven years without any problems.

She started work at 8.00 am, had a 15 minute break at 10.30 am, half an hour for lunch, 15 minutes break in the afternoon and usually finished at about 5.00 pm and doing a five day week.

Her work was essentially that of a weaver. She grasped a cotton thread, and, by a vigorous extension movement at the wrist whilst holding the thread between the thumb and forefinger, she drew it towards her before allowing the bobbin to pull the thread back, flexing her wrist, before, again with the extension of the wrist, the whole procedure was repeated.

Only the dominant right hand was used, the left hand being employed in guiding the thread on the bobbin.

The weaving manoeuvre took place about 50 times every minute a total of 3,000 times an hour and over 20,000 movements during the working day.

It was necessary to stand up in order to control the bobbins and she often complained to management that she would like to have had some form of job rotation. This however, was not forthcoming, nor were her complaints of backache and sore feet from standing on the York stone flagged floor in the mill taken seriously.

Although she was not happy with the boredom and repetitive nature of the work jobs were difficult to come by in the area in which she lived, and she had two children and an invalid husband, relying on her so she put up with the problems.

The mill was then sold to an international company who stated that, following the end of the summer holidays – during which the entire mill closed down – there would be a bonus system coming into effect but there would also be redundancies among the weaving staff.

When Mrs Pitt returned from holiday she found she was expected to increase her output which meant that instead of 50 she would need to do about 55 flexion/extension movements of the right hand a minute if she were to achieve the bonus. It was also made clear that those that did not reach the bonus number would be considered for redundancy.

Mrs Pitt was able to increase her output by reducing her work breaks and pushing herself a bit harder. There were no problems for the two months and then she started to get aches and pains over the right radial styloid. She persevered with the work but went to her GP who advised her to take painkillers during the working day. She did this but nevertheless started to get a painful swelling at the base of the right thumb which became worse in spite of the painkilling drugs. She saw the works' doctor who suggested a variation in the type of work she was doing. This suggestion was not taken up by management and, although she had a week's sick leave, when she returned she was back on the same job.

The pain then came on within an hour of her starting the working day and was particularly bad when she abducted the thumb. She persevered but after a further three weeks she found she was unable to meet the bonus requirements and was made redundant.

When examined by a consultant rheumatologist she was found to have pain over the radial styloid and there was tenderness over the pollicis brevis and abductor pollicis longus tendons. He diagnosed de Quervain's tenovaginitis and injected the area with steroids. This was repeated on three occasions with only short term benefit but, finally, surgical decompression gave her considerable improvement.

She was unable to return to her previous job and when seen she was looking for work outside the textile industry.

The medical opinion was that, on the balance of probabilities, Mrs Pitt had a work related upper limb disorder manifesting itself as a de Quervain's tenovaginitis of the tendons of extensor pollicis brevis and abductor pollicis longus muscles.[54]

The lawyers were not convinced it would be possible to prove causation and, as the Trade Union advisers had to take a similar view, the action against the employers was not pursued.

## Vibration White Finger in a Gas Fitter

Mr Sims was a 38 year old fitter who had been working for a gas servicing company without problems for about four years. For much of the time he was using a hand held percussive hammer to assist in the laying of new gas pipes. The hammer weighed about 10 lbs and although it is not known how many vibrations it put out Mr Sims said it issued a high powered constant vibrating hum which suggested an output in excess of 1,000 vibrations per minute.

The hammer was usually held in the left hand, guided by the right, and was often in use for much of the day. After about four years he noticed the index finger on the left hand was inclined to be painful, with pins and needles, particularly in cold weather, and was excessively cold even in hot weather.

He did not report these symptoms to management as he did not think it was of any great significance but gradually the third and forth fingers on the left and then the thumb on the right hand became involved and the fingers became white or blanched.

There was also a loss of sensation in his fingers when using the hammer which would persist even after he had stopped using the hammer at the end of the day but improved if he put his hands in warm water.

At first his hand problems were worse in winter or in cold weather and improved when he was on holiday, when he wore gloves, or when he was spending only short periods using the percussion hammer. Gradually however, the condition worsened and after about seven years it was present even during the warm summer days and did not go away at night or on holiday.

He had finally reported the condition to the gas company medical officer who thought there was some form of peripheral vascular problem and advised various ways of continuing with his work whilst protecting his hands. This failed to help the situation and it became very difficult for Mr Sims to do many of the routine jobs around the house as he lacked sensation in his fingers. He was therefore, referred to a consultant in occupational medicine who diagnosed vibration white finger.

The consultant advised Mr Sims to give up his job as otherwise his condition would deteriorate further. He did so, has been unable to work in the gas industry since that time, and the problems with his fingers and thumb persist.

The vibration white finger syndrome took about eight years to develop from its first appearance until he was unable to continue with his job as a gas fitter.

*Discussion*

Vibration white finger has been known since the nineteenth century as a problem in the use of vibrating tools. It was thought to be a type of Raynaud's phenomena in which, as a result of the vibration of the tools impairing the nerves which controls the blood vessels, there was a reduction in the amount of blood and circulating oxygen to the hands.

This condition has appeared frequently in the history of commerce and industry particularly where there is the need for vibrating tools or machines such as hammers, chain saws, metal cleaners and percussion drills. This has led to a clear understanding of the dangers of the vibrating tool and to that end it is now one of the prescribed industrial diseases (A11).

Mr Sims was one of a number of men in his work team who developed vibration white finger and they all had in common the use of the percussion hammer.

A substantial financial settlement was agreed out of Court largely based on the fact that the condition is incurable and at the age of 42 Mr Sims' job opportunities, and thus his income, would be adversely affected for the remainder of his life as a result of the irreversible changes which the use of the vibrating tools had brought about in his hands.

## Doffer's Elbow (Epicondylitis) in a Chemical Manufacturing Worker

Mr Steel worked for a chemical manufacturing company for 23 years before taking early retirement on medical grounds. As a result of the nature of his work he developed a condition known locally as 'Doffer's Elbows' which is a type of epicondylitis.

'Doffing' means unloading and when doffing the men would adopted a crouching position on steps in a type of inspection pit beneath a machine. They would then each lift an 8 pound nylon bobbin by a narrow rim at the top – using only all the finger tips of the left hand – and push the bobbin up into a box. At the same time the right hand was unloading 'cakes', a type of chemical, into the machine.

This was arduous and repetitive work throughout the day. There were six machines each of which had 140 bobbins and the six were worked by three men, each man thus lifted many hundreds of pounds of bobbins and 'cakes' during a shift mainly using the hands and forearms. It was this simultaneous loading and unloading which made such demands on the elbows.

During the ten years previous to his leaving the company the speed, weight and repetitive nature of the doffing work increased in line with various productivity agreements.

Mr Steel started having problems after twelve years doffing and his GP records demonstrate he was seen for a condition which was first described as tennis elbow. The condition apparently became unbearable in April 1994 when 'whilst loading cakes I felt pain in my shoulder'. He was given two weeks off but when he returned to work he continued to have acute pain particularly in the right arm and right shoulder. Epicondylitis and capsulitis was diagnosed, but x-rays of the right shoulder revealed little of significance and he was referred for physiotherapy – which gave him no relief.

He describes very graphically how during his 23 years at the chemical factory doffer's elbow was suffered by all the doffers to one degree or another. With the advent of the pain in the elbows it was apparently common for there to be guarding or favouring of one or other of the arms which leads to pain in the shoulders. This combination of elbow and shoulder pain was suffered by all the doffers.

He was on light duties during the final three years of his time at the chemical manufacturing plant but the chronic pain in both elbows and the right shoulder, finally became too much for him and he took early retirement.

He cannot now do many of the routine domestic jobs around the house and garden without pain. He is restricted when cleaning his car, doing home decorating, using a chisel for wood turning, or, of he can manage to carry out these activities, it is only in a restricted way and associated with pain, particularly in his right shoulder. He cannot easily straighten our his arms which makes carrying shopping bags and writing difficult. There is a loss of sensation in his fingers. Holding up his arms when driving causes pain and as a result he has to be driven by his wife. At the age of 61 he knows he will never again be in gainful employment.

He worked what is described as a 'continental shift system' – that is 2.00 am to 2.00 pm for three days and then 2.00 pm to 10.00 pm and 10.00 pm to 6.00 pm. He wore ear muffs whilst working and was given a noise allowance. He had adequate breaks during his work shifts.

On examination there was pain on movement of the elbows, at the common extensor origin. Shrugging the shoulders produced an acute pain in the right shoulder as did all movements of the right arm – particularly abduction – due to a rotator cuff syndrome.

*Discussion*

As a result of the injury to his elbows Mr Steel favoured his forearms and thus placed extra musculo-skeletal pressures on his right shoulder. The shoulder pain is therefore, secondary to the elbow problems and is a supraspinatus tendonitis or a rotator cuff syndrome. These conditions have arisen directly from the repetitive awkward position he was forced to adopt and to the repetitive nature of the doffing work. The end result was that the chronic epicondylitis caused excessive stresses to be placed also on the acromio-clavicular joint and the soft tissues surrounding the right shoulder.

*Prognosis*

Mr Steel was justified in retiring early as by then he had three years in the 'monitoring unit' – which was essentially a means of offering him light employment. Yet at the end of those three years he was still suffering incapacitating pains in his elbows and right shoulder.

Mr Steel has now had doffer's elbow, to one degree or another, for more than eight years and it is likely he will continue to have long term problems.

*Opinion*

Mr Steel has suffered, and is suffering from, a work related upper limb disorder manifesting itself as bi-lateral epicondylitis and injury to the soft tissues of the right shoulder and known as 'Doffer's Elbows'.

This action was settled out of Court and Mr Steel received £30,000.

## Tenosynovitis in a Pottery Worker

Mrs Jackson worked in various parts of the Stoke-On-Trent pottery industry for much of her adult life and, until 1994, had suffered only minor aches and pains as a result of the often heavy and repetitive nature of the pottery manufacturing procedures.

In 1994 she was working as a lithographer. A lithographer applies coloured or decorative transfers on to a pottery surface before it is fired in the kiln to give a permanent finish. Mrs Jackson was an experienced lithographer and capable of working on a wide variety of pottery – cups, mugs, teapots, tureens – but for the benefit of this report the working arrangements involved in the lithography of mugs alone will be considered.

By 1994 Mrs Jackson had been at the factory for about five years and, during a working shift was capable of processing 70 to 75 dozen mugs. She is right handed and both hands were continuously involved in the working procedures. She would lift a mug with her left hand, position it on the machine.

In February 1994 a more efficient machine was introduced to the factory which allowed a greatly increased throughput of mugs. As a result of this automation some workers were made redundant, others were moved to different jobs, but Mrs Jackson was retained to work the new machines. So effective was this machine that output increased from 70 dozen to 425 dozen mugs per shift. Whilst much of this increase was as a result of the efficiency of the machine nevertheless each mug had to be handled at least twice which led to an enormous –

probably six fold – increase in the number of repetitive movements carried out by Mrs Jackson's hands in the course of an eight hour shift. Management was unsympathetic to her complaints, or requests for job rotation, and there was ever present threat of redundancy.

By May 1994 the increased demands made upon the soft tissues of her hands and arms by these repetitive movements had resulted in the onset of pain, which, initially came on at the end of the working day and lasting into the evening. This pain gradually extended its domain, interrupting her sleeping patterns, and then started to affect her working capabilities. The pain was accompanied by swelling, tingling and tremor in both hands which finally persisted day and night. She had a two week holiday at the end of June and early July 1994 which allowed some recovery but as soon as she returned to work and was forced to accept the same working conditions the pain started again and increased in intensity until by August 1994 she was unable to continue working on the assembly line and was laid off. Her contract was terminated in March 1995.

There are many references in the GP and hospital notes to the hand and arms problems – and reactive depression – and to physiotherapy being of little benefit. She went before the Medical Appeal Tribunal in February 1996 whose decision was that she was suffering from 'Prescribed Disease A8 Tenosynovitis'.

*Current Problems*

If she carries out any form of heavy work such as hoovering or carrying shopping bags the back of her forearms swell and there is pain along the extensor tendons. The power and sensitivity in her hands has been reduced; she states 'they don't feel like my own hands'. She is thus unable to do many of the routine jobs around the house particularly if they involve lifting kettles, crockery or saucepans as she is in danger of dropping them. Shopping has to be done by her husband

and she can no longer do jobs in the garden, and the loss of sensation in the fingers has meant that sewing and knitting are difficult.

*On Examination of the Musculo-Skeletal System*

The power was reduced in both hands, there was loss of muscle bulk in the hypothenar eminence, and the small muscles of the back of the hands appeared to be poorly developed.

There were no abnormalities of movement in the hands or arms although vigorous pronation and supination provoked pain in the forearms, particularly in the forearm extensors.

All reflexes in the arms were brisk and there was some loss of sensation at the tips of all the fingers which did not conform to any particular nerve distribution – neither median or ulnar.

At the time of examination there was no forearm swelling, nor crepitus.

*Discussion*

Mrs Jackson carried out many repetitive and arduous tasks in the pottery industry during the 24 years of her working life without any significant problems until, in February 1994, she was put in charge of a new machine which allowed a greatly increased throughput of mugs. The increased output and the consequential increase in the number of repetitive movements of the hands and forearms led, within three months, to the onset of pins and needles in the fingers, swelling in both hands, pain on the back of the hands radiating into the forearms, with tremor and loss of power in the hands. As a result of these problems she was unable to continue working and she lost her job.

She was assessed by the DSS in February 1996 who diagnosed tenosynovitis as did her GP who saw her during the acute phase of the condition. However, the fact that when seen in 1997 she stilled suffered problems would suggest there was also an element of non specific pain syndrome.

*Prognosis*
It is likely that if Mrs Jackson avoids those repetitive activities and movements which provoke the aches and pains in the hands and forearms, there could be some gradual long term improvement.

*Opinion*
Mrs Jackson has a work related condition of the upper limbs manifesting itself as tenosynovitis and non specific pain syndrome of the forearm extensors and, in particular, the extensor carpi ulnaris, extensor digiti minimi and extensor digitorum muscles.

This action was settled out of Court for £26,000.

## Non Specific Pain Syndrome in a Printing Machine Operator

Mrs Henderson is aged 45 and between 1988 and March 1997 she worked as a machine operator processing pottery figures, without, for the first eight years, any problems with her hands or arms.

In November 1996 her working procedures involved picking up a figure with her right – dominant – hand using all fingers and thumb in a gripping, pinching action associated with flexion and extension movements at the wrists, as she positioned the figure on the jig of the machine in front of her. The jig was held stationary in the centre whilst the machine was in constant rotation around it printing designs on to the pottery. When the printing was finished Mrs Henderson would lift the figure from the jig with her left hand, again involving all fingers, thumb and wrist movements, to move it to a tray on the left – to avoid the paint being smeared. At the same time her right hand was picking up another figurine from the box to her right and replacing it for the painted one. She was seated in a chair which gave her inadequate support and she needed to constantly lean forward to control the procedures.

Her hours of work were 8.00 am to 4.30 pm, with a half hour unpaid lunch break, and 15 minutes paid breaks at 10.00 am and 3.00 pm. Otherwise she was operating the machine throughout the working day – often into overtime.

There were about 15 machines of three basic types in the factory and 24 women would rotate between them so as not – in theory – to spend more than two hours on the more demanding machines. When they were less busy they might rotate jobs on a daily basis.

She was expected to place 12 to 14 figurines on to the jig every minute and, at times when the he rate of production was increased, this represented as many as 1,000 units per hour.

Management was clearly aware of the danger to their employees of failing to ring the changes on their more repetitive activities and, until November 1996 – when a less experienced manager took over – there appears to have been no problems on the shop floor.

Until November 1996 Mrs Henderson had been working the printing machine in tandem with another women one of whom would place the figure on the jig and the other would take it off after it was painted and move it to the tray. This trouble free policy then changed and, in spite of her protests, Mrs Henderson was forced to manage the machine single handed which, effectively, meant a doubling of her work load. The new management also had innovative ideas about improving the throughput and thus the number of figures she needed to handle was increased to as many as 18 units per minute.

Thus in the Autumn of 1996 she was disadvantaged in three ways. Forced to work the machine herself, required to accept a greatly increased work load; and subject to abuse from the shop floor when she complained to the unhelpful management. She was thus under considerable pressure both physically and psychologically.

The machines were designed in a way which made greater use on the left arm and in about December /January 1996/97 she started to develop pains in the left shoulder and left arm and pins and needles in all the left fingers and thumb. By February 1997 she had developed similar aches and pains in the right shoulder, arm and hand. These symptoms initially came on in the afternoon and persisted into the evening but within a few weeks they were present when she reported to work in the morning and kept her awake at night.

She first realised she had a real problem when she was on the bus and was unable to grip the hand hold and a friend needed to assist her off the bus and take her home.

She therefore, went to see her general practitioner who thought her problems were work related and she was given two weeks away from the factory. She felt a little better for having the break but the pains persisted when she returned to work and to the same machine and under the same psychological pressures.

She needed the income so she took pain killers which allowed her to continue working until August 1997 when she was forced to hand in her notice as she found it too difficult to continue as she was in constant pain and was unable to keep up the required output.

*Current Problems*

There has been some improvement since she gave up work but the problems return as soon as she makes any demanding use of her hands. She has pain in both arms, neck and back, and develops pain at night if she lies on her left side. As a result of this she has difficulty with many of the routine social and domestic activities, hoovering or any work involving pushing or pulling manoeuvres are particularly difficult, she has dropped glasses and cups due to the weakness of her hands and is concerned about holding kettles and saucepans; turning taps or knobs or working tin openers, causes pain and she cannot carry any weight of significance.

She no longer has the confidence to drive her car as she lacks the strength to put on the hand brake.

As a result of having to give up her job her relationship with her husband has been put under strain and she has become depressed, having never been so previously, and has been treated with anti-depressants.

The GP and other records show she had no problems with her arms or shoulders until the Spring of 1997 and suggest her problems are work related and had developed over the previous few months.

> 'On examination she was a slim ectomorphic woman. She can bend down and touch her toes being limited by some pain in the thoracic spine. All movements of the head and neck – flexion, extension and moving left and right – cause pain in the cervical spine. Abduction of the arms above the head are achieved with some difficulty as is putting her hands separately behind her back to touch her bra strap.'

Her hands show no loss of power but there appears to have been some loss of muscle bulk in both hands – although being of a slim build this might not be of any significance.

She indicated the pins and needles as being present in all fingers but Tinel's and Phelan's tests for carpal tunnel syndrome were negative. There is no limitation in movement in all the fingers and the wrists, and there was no evidence of epicondylitis or nerve entrapment.

Shrugging the shoulders causes some pain in the cervical spine as does palpation over the cervical vertebrae and she has tender trigger points in the trapezius muscle on palpation.

*Discussion*

Mrs Henderson worked for over eight years in the pottery industry without any problems until in the Autumn of 1996 there was a change in management and working policies. She was then forced to work single handed at a machine which had previously required two women; management who were unsympathetic to her complaints or to requests for job rotation and, in fact, increased her expected output from 14 to 18 units per minute.

The result of this was that she was carrying out repetitive movements involving the muscles of the thumb and fingers and the flexors and extensors or the forearms – whilst siting in a hunched position at the work station – as many as 6,000 to 7,000 times in a working day – and in an oppressive working atmosphere.

Mrs Henderson was confronted with many of the undesirable working conditions which are known to bring about a work related upper limb disorder. These involve rapid repetitive movements as part of the working procedures, awkward working positions, poor workplace tool and equipment design, excessive work rates, lack of job variation, inadequate rest breaks, process lines being speeded up, overbearing supervision, lack of individual control over the working process and changes in the work process. She also took pain killers which allowed her to continue to work – but which changed and acute into chronic condition.

*Prognosis*

It is possible that there will be some improvement if she avoids those activities of a repetitive nature which brought on the problems in the first place. She will not be able to return to any form of factory work which involves repetitive activities and she would be wise to think of some form of re-training.

*Opinion*
Mrs Henderson has suffered a work related upper limb disorder manifesting itself as a non specific pain syndrome and arising out of the nature of her work during the period November 1996 to March 1997.

This action is in the hands of the solicitors.

## Non Specific Pain Syndrome in a Factory Worker

Mrs James first joined an engineering company in 1986 and started working in the plating shop. At that time the assembly line was manned by eight women but, over the years, the number was gradually reduced to four – but with no reduction in the expected work output. It was shortly after the work force was reduced to four (1993) that she started to develop pains in the right hand and arm. The works' medical documentation faithfully records these developments and there is no suggestion that her problems were otherwise than work related. A diagnosis of right de Quervain's tenosynovitis was made and, specifically, the abductor and extensor muscles – particularly those involving the right thumb – were incriminated. She was treated with tubi-grip, given time off work and advised to see her GP. She was also questioned as to the number and type of pain killers she was taking and advised to try and do without them.

Between March 1993 and September 1994 there are about 30 entries in the works' medical records clearly recording the progress of her musculo-skeletal problems particularly in the right arm. At no time was there any suggestion that the problems were not work related.

In September 1994 the records state:

> 'There is today clinical evidence of bi-lateral tennis elbow and de Quervain's tenosynovitis. She is not

> suitable for the plating shop. She can do work which is not too arduous or repetitive. If any job fits these criteria she should move there otherwise she should be considered unemployable.'

There was thus about a two year period between the onset off the right arm problems and her being forced to give up work. During this period she saw a number of doctors, various investigations were carried out, a number of provisional diagnoses were made, and treatments were initiated – none of which were of any significant benefit to her.[54]

In November 1996 Mrs James was awarded Industrial Injuries Disablement Benefit in respect of prescribed tenosynovitis at a rate of 20%.

*Working Procedures*

Mrs James identified photographs in an ergonomist's report showing the jigs and other machinery involved in her day to day activities. She then demonstrated, using both hands, the nature of the movements involved and the rapidity with which these movements were carried out. The ergonomist's report demonstrates that in a typical day she handled about 4,000 components, each of which required loading and unloading from the jig to a total of about 8,000 manual manipulations. This is equivalent to about 1,000 movements per hour or one every three or four seconds throughout the working day.

Because of the manpower reduction in the plating shop Mrs James effectively, over a period of years, needed to double her labours in order to keep up with an output which was previously achieved by twice as many women.

The Health & Safety Executive Publication *Work Related Upper Limb Disorders* lists four predisposing conditions likely to cause a work related upper limb disorder; the application of an undesirable manual Force, the Frequency and Duration of Movements, and Posture.

When applying these criteria to Mrs James' working conditions it is clear she was probably at risk from all four factors. She needed to apply significant force when attaching the components to the jigs, the frequency and duration of the activity was increased over the years and she needed to adopt an undesirable working posture.

Nor did her hours of work allow for sufficient rest breaks. She worked from 7.45 am to 4.15 pm five days a week but was given only a 10 minute break in the morning and half an hour break at lunch time – and yet needed to catch up on the work which had accumulated during these breaks. There was no break in the afternoon which meant a long period of unrelieved activity.

There was a strong emphasis in her working procedures on the use of the thumb and the first finger in a gripping movement. It is thus significant that the main muscles involved in this movement – abductor pollicis longus and extensor pollicis brevis – are those incriminated in de Quervain's tenosynovitis – which appears to have been a diagnosis from the very beginning.

*Current Complaints*

When seen there had been some improvement over the previous two years but the pain persists in the hands and the elbows and any form of heavy work such as hoovering, washing up, cleaning windows, carrying heavy shopping bags, or preparing vegetables is likely over the following few hours, to cause swelling of the hands and forearms.

She has learnt to pace herself and to adjust her activities, where possible, to avoid problems – and making more use of the left hand helps to protect the right.

On examination there is no limitation or pain on flexion, extension medial and lateral rotation of the neck and flexion, extension, supination and pronation at the wrists is achieved without difficulty. There is no evidence of tenosynovitis, de Quervain's tenosynovitis or carpal tunnel syndrome and, at the elbows, there is no pain on palpation of the medial and lateral epicondyles (golfer's or tennis elbow).

There is however, some puffiness at the base of the right thumb and to a lesser extent at the base of the left thumb and she indicates the pain as being present along the line of the extensor muscle to the thumb and index finger.

*Discussion*

Mrs James worked for nearly 7 years without any significant problems in her upper limbs. There was then a gradual reduction in the plating department work force which led to a doubling in the amount of heavy repetitive work she needed to carry out many thousands of times a day, mainly using the extensor and flexor muscles of the right hand.

With the increased workload she stared to develop aches and pains in her hands and arms which are faithfully recorded for two and a half years in the works' medical records. It is clear that although a number off diagnoses were considered by the various doctors involved it was apparently never in question that the cause of her problems was work related.

She finally found it impossible to continue and in 1996 she was discharged on medical grounds and has not worked since.

When seen there were no signs of any of the prescribed industrial diseases but the medical history is clearly of a work related soft tissue condition which has changed its presentation over the past three or four years. There was no signs of de Quervain's or any other type of tenosynovitis, the epicondylitis was no longer present, and the previous shoulder and neck problems had resolved with rest.

However, it is clear that a residual pathology remains which manifests itself particularly as aching and swelling of the right hand when she carries out any form or heavy or repetitive work.

*Prognosis*

The hand and arm problems appear to have reached a plateau but if she were to return to any form of repetitive work involving the hands, then the problem would return.

Re-training may well be the only answer as she is only 37 and some form of long term employment will be essential.

*Opinion*

Mrs James has a work related upper limb disorder now manifesting as a non-specific pain syndrome and arising out of the nature of her work and, in particular, the period of intense activity when the labour force in the plating department was reduced from eight to fours.

The legal action continues.

# Glossary

## INTRODUCTION

Something strange can come over medical practitioners when they start to write about WRULDs. Doctors who would never be imprecise when writing about tuberculosis, cancer, diabetes or other disease processes often retreat into abstruse verbiage when writing about WRULDs and not only use words and phrases which are meaningless to many of their colleagues – never mind the layman – but they even invent new ones. This has many disadvantages, not least the difficulty of comparing like with like and thus the inhibiting effect this has on epidemiological studies.

In an attempt to penetrate this obfuscation I have compiled a list of the terms used in WRULD reports and publications and, where possible, I have attempted to explain their meaning.

**Abnormal Illness Behaviour** – This has already achieved the acronym AIB and was first described by Powlowski in 1969 as the 'persistence of an inappropriate maladaptive mode of perceiving, evaluating, and acting in relation to one's state of health'. The physical signs were said to include wide spread non-anatomic tenderness and the patients concerned magnified their pain using emotive terms. The abnormal behaviour was thought to be related to the anticipation of financial gain or some form of compensation.

**Acromio-Clavicular Syndrome** – Injury to, or overuse of, the arm can cause persistent upward displacement of the lateral end of the clavicle with pain, worse during full elevation of the arm.

**Adverse Neural Tension** – This is a test often used by physiotherapists to differentiate between pain arising in the nerve roots from that arising in the soft tissues. Specifically it is used to differentiate between pain arising in the cervical nerve roots, and brachial plexus, and pain arising from the muscle bursae and joint capsule in the neck and shoulders.

**Algodystrophy** – See Reflex Sympathetic Dystrophy.

**Allodynia** – This is the term given to the hypersensitivity reaction to touch and gentle palpation. The term Allopathia is sometimes used if the hypersensitivity is such as to lead to feelings of burning, electric shocks and excessive pins and needles.

**Anatomical Orientation** – To help in the descriptions of an anatomical structure or region of the body certain terms are used that have an agreed interpretation. The *Anatomical Position* is one in which the person stands upright, feet together, eyes looking forward, arms straight along the side of the body with the palms of the hands directed forwards. The front of the body is called the *Anterior* surface and the back is called the *Posterior* surface. *Ventral* and *Dorsal* are also used to describe the front and the back.

Higher structures are *Superior* and lower structures are *Inferior*. *Median* structures are in the midline of the body or a limb. *Medial* means nearer to the midline and Lateral means further away from the midline

A *Sagittal* plane passes vertically anteroposteriorly through the body and forward movements in this plane are called *Flexion* and backward movements are *Extension*. A vertical plane at right angles to the sagittal is called a *Coronal* plane and movements of joints in this plane are *Abduction* or away from, and *Adduction* towards the midline. Rotation can occur in certain joints along a longitudinal axis.

**Anterior Interosseous Syndrome** – This syndrome is due to pressure over the anterior interosseous nerve in the upper arm and leads to weakness of flexion of the terminal digit of the index finger and thumb demonstrated as loss of normal pinch.

**Arcade of Frohse** – This is part of the tendinous/membranous origin of the supinator muscle at the lateral epicondyle of the humerus (outer aspect of the elbow). The posterior interosseous nerve (a branch of the radial nerve) passes between the superficial and deep parts of the supinator muscle where it may be trapped causing pain. (See Radial Tunnel Syndrome).

**Arthropathy** – Any joint pain.

**Arthroscopy** – Examination of the interior of a joint with an arthroscope.

**Arthroplasty** – Plastic surgery of a joint, or the formation of moveable joints.

**Barre-Lieou Syndrome** – A syndrome of pains in the upper neck, headaches, vertigo, diplopia, tinnitus, tempro-mandibular – joint and unspecific facial – pains possibly arising in the cervical spine.

**Beat Hand** – Subcutaneous cellulitis of the hand or inflammation of the bursae (synovial lined sacs) leading to bursitis in the hands of miners or workers with picks and shovels. Similar inflammatory conditions are produced in the elbows and knees (beat elbow and beat knee). All are prescribed industrial diseases.

**Bicipital Tendonitis** – This complaint is characterised by pain in the front of the shoulder worsening on active use of the arm and is thought to be caused by excessive use of the shoulder joint. It is also known as 'tenosynovitis of the long tendon of the biceps' and is characterised by pain and local tenderness in the region of the bicipital groove of the humerus and the long tendon of the biceps. It is thought to be caused by friction and irritation of the tendon in its groove.

**Brachial Plexus** – The roots of the brachial plexus are largely formed from the union of the anterior primary rami of the lower four cervical nerves and the greater part of the anterior primary ramus of the first thoracic nerve. The plexus lies within the axilla and may be incriminated in many WRULD's.

**Brachialgia** – Pain in the arm or arms.

**Brachialgia Statica Paraesthetica** – Painful pins and needles in the arms when asleep due to compression of the blood vessels.

**Brachial Plexus Tension Test** – This is similar to the neural tension test in that it helps to distinguish between shoulder and arm pain due to irritation of the nerve roots and that due to pain arising from the soft tissues of the shoulder region.

**Bursitis** – Bursitis is inflammation or infection of the bursae which surround joints such as at the patella (housemaids' knee) the metatarsal head (bunion), the hand (beat hand).

**Carpal Tunnel Syndrome** – This is a common cause of discomfort in the hand especially in middle aged or elderly women. It is caused by pressure on the median nerve as it passes from the forearm into the hand within the firm walled carpal tunnel. The pressure produces a tingling, numbness or discomfort in the radial fingers (outer three and a half digits) and there is a feeling of clumsiness in carrying out fine movements such as those involved in sewing. The symptoms and signs vary with the degree and duration of the compression of the median nerve. It is thought that repeated flexion and extension at the wrist – as is common in various work related activities – can cause fluid to accumulate and put pressure on the median nerve causing the typical carpal tunnel syndrome. There are however, other causes of neurological disturbances in the hand including those arising in the neck, from interference with the brachial plexus, and lesions of the median nerve elsewhere in its anatomical course. Such diseases as muscular dystrophy and syringomyelia may also cause similar neurological disturbance.

**Cervical Spondylosis**
This is osteoarthritis of the cervical spine. Degenerative changes in the cervical spine are very common and although they may be due to injury – such as whiplash – they are most commonly due to the aging process. The condition is often symptomless, but it may be a cause of aching pain in the neck or trapezius muscles. Less often there is pressure on the nerve roots leading to radiating pain along the course of the affected nerve or nerves and to 'tingling' or 'pins or needles' in the hand.

**CMC Joint** – Carpometacarpal joint.

**Cognitive Therapy** – A type of psychological therapy practised in some pain clinics which can allow patients to come to terms with, and accept, chronic pain.

**Compensation** – An award made by a court in compensation for, amongst other things, personal injury sustained as a result of occupational activities.

**Compensation Neurosis** – This is also known as 'accident neurosis' or 'litigation neurosis' terms which reflect the view that patients adapt or exaggerate their symptoms, and physical signs if they are present, in an effort to increase the possibility of compensation – or to gain in some other manner.

**Constructive Dismissal** – A case for constructive dismissal could be made out if an employer failed to respond to complaints about, for example, unsatisfactory working conditions thus causing a work related upper limb disorder which led to the employee having to give up his work.

**Constitutional** – This is a term used when a medical condition is thought not to be due to an occupational factor but due to some physical or physiological characteristic specific to the person concerned which makes them more vulnerable than normal to a precipitating factor. This may indeed be true, as a group of workers exposed to the same adverse working conditions may respond in quite different ways, reflecting the inherent variability of mankind. Alternatively a constitutional factor may bring about a more exacerbated response to an occupational situation. On the other hand the phrase 'constitutional' may be used when the medical practitioner is inexperienced or prejudiced.

**Conversion Disorder** – This is one of the vague psychological terms used, and often in a very unspecific way, to describe the psychological responses to WRULDs.

**Conversion Hysteria** – A diagnosis which was put forward in Australia to explain the symptoms of what later became known as 'RSI'. It was used in the UK in 1998 in the *Pickford* v. *ICI* Action but it was proved at trial that this medical phenomena only arises where the individual has knowledge of the risks of RSI.

**Craft Palsy or Craft Cramps** – These are the old names of some of the conditions which today would be called work related upper limb disorders or overuse syndromes.

**Cramp of the Hand** – A prescribed industrial disease (A4). See Clinical Syndromes.

**Crepitus** – When palpating over a tendon a grating feeling and tenderness is indicative of inflammation within the synovial sheath, i.e. tenosynovitis.

**de Quervain's Stenosing Tenovaginitis** – This is a type of tenosynovitis of the tendons of the muscles of the thumb as they pass into the wrist. The pain is over the styloid process of the radius and there is a palpable nodule in the course of the abductor pollicus longus and extensor pollicus brevis tendons. This is a similar condition to trigger finger. The cause is unknown but is often associated with repetitive activities involving much use of the thumb and forefinger and wrists such as wringing clothes, working at machines or on assembly lines.

**Disablement Benefit** – Disablement Benefit can be paid by the DSS to those people suffering from industrial disease as prescribed by the Industrial Injuries Advisory Council.

**Dupuytren's Contracture** – This is a condition characterised by a flexion contracture of one or more of the fingers due to thickening and shortening of the palmar aponeurosis (thin fibrous sheet of tissue on the palm of the hand). The flexion is much more common in men than in women and often both hands are affected. The other sign is a small thickened nodule in the mid palm opposite the base of the ring finger. The area thickened gradually spreads from this point giving rise eventually to firm cord like bands that extend into the ring or little finger preventing full extension of the metacarpal-phalangeal, and the proximal inter-phalangeal joints. The flexion deformity becomes progressively worse over the course of months or years and surgery may be necessary.

**Dysaethesia** – Insensitivity or derangement of sensation or the senses.

**Dystonic Phenomena** – These may manifest itself as poor coordination, cramps, fatigue on repetitive movements and loss of fine movements. There may be motor weakness but no significant muscle wasting.

**Dysarthrosis** – Deformity or malformation of a joint.

**Dysthymic** – Depressed in spirits or dejected.

**Dyschiria** – Derangement of the power to tell which arm (or other part of the body) has been touched.

**Dyscrasia** – A term formerly used to indicate an abnormal mixture of the four humours but in modern usage is roughly synonymous with 'disease' or 'pathologic condition'

**Dysphoria** – A state of unpleasant mood alternation – which can be drug induced.

**Dystrophy** – Disorders arising from genetic abnormalities or faulty nutrition and affecting muscle groups, i.e. the muscular dystrophies.

**Dyskinesia** – Distortion or impairment of voluntary movements as in spasm or tic.

**Endorphins** – These morphine like substances are produced on exercise and have a direct action on the brain giving a sense of euphoria.

**Enthesitis** – Inflammation of the muscular or tendinous attachment to bone.

**Entheses** – The entheses are the insertions into bone of collagenous structures such as tendons, ligaments and articular capsules. The entheses are subjected to heavy loads and it is probably repeated stresses that cause the characteristic changes or abnormalities in the entheses which are called enthesopathies.

**Enthesopathies** – As far as work related upper limb disorders are concerned the most common enthesopathies are the tennis and golfer's elbows (where the tendons are inserted into the lateral epicondyle and medial epicondyle) leading to epicondylitis. Others are the supraspinatus tendinitis, and the abductor longus tendinitis. The long tendon of the biceps, supraspinatus tendon, and the extensor pollicis longus are three examples of tendons which are prone to rupture without violent stress or injury.

**Epicondylitis** – This is characterised by pain in the lateral or medial aspect of the elbow often radiating down into the forearm. It is due to inflammation caused by strain of the forearm extensor or flexor muscles at their point of origin. Epicondylitis appears under many names such as tenniselbow, golfer's elbow, javelin thrower's arm, but many occupational jobs involving hammering or lifting with outstretched fingers under pressure may bring about this typical clinical picture.

**Epistemological** – Epistemology is the science which deals with the origin, method and validity of knowledge.

**Ergonomics** – The application of strict engineering and scientific principles to the design of the work place and the work place equipment, tools, machinery, seats and furniture. 'Fitting the worker to the job and the job to the worker.'

**Expert Witness** – The function of an expert witness is to assist the Court in coming to a conclusion. It is not the function of an expert witness to be biased one way or another. He should be an expert in his field and prepared to give his opinion dispassionately – no matter who is paying his fee. The expert witness should be able to act either for the Plaintiff or the Defendant being there merely to put forward the facts to allow the Court to come to its own conclusion based on those facts.

> *It would be off no assistance to the Courts if doctors were encouraged to abandon their professional approach and write reports designed to achieve particular objectives, at the behest of the patient or anyone else.*
>
> *Noble* v. *Robert Thompson* 1979

**Fibromyalgia** – This is a rather unspecific condition bearing little difference to fibrositis and manifesting itself as diffuse musculoskeletal aching associated with tender points in the neck and shoulders. It may bear many resemblances to the old fashioned phrase 'lumbago'.

**Finkelstein's Test** – A test for de Quervain's tenovaginitis in which there is pain on ulnar deviation of the clenched fist when the thumb is folded into the palm of the hand.

**Flick Test** – Patients suffering from carpal tunnel syndrome may sometimes gain symptomatic relief by a rapid flick of the hand

**Focal Dystonia** – See Dystonic Phenomena.

**Frozen Shoulder** – This is characterised by aches and pains in the shoulder and upper arm, of spontaneous or gradual onset associated with impairment of movement. The cause is not understood but is probably related to repetitive use, or misuse, of the shoulder joint which may lead to loss of resilience of the joint capsule.

**Ganglion** – This is the commonest cystic swelling at the back of the wrist and can be seen in adults of any age. On examination the swelling may be soft and cystic but it can also be quite tense and easily mistaken for a bony prominence. It is harmless and in the absence of pain or complications, due to pressure on to an underlying nerve, it is probably best left untreated.

**Gate Control Theory of Pain** – This provides the physiological basis for an explanation of the observed pain phenomena and the effective and cognitive aspects of pain. The transmission of afferent nerve impulses is considered to be modulated at spinal dorsal horn level by a gating mechanism. Several interacting neural systems, including those from higher centres ('beyond the gate') have an excitatory or inhibitory function at the gate. When neural transmission reaches a critical level, and the gate is opened, a complex pattern of responses results in the experience and manifestations of pain.

**Gowers, Sir William** – Sir William Gowers, Consultant Neurologist, University College London, 1845–1915 wrote on writer's cramp and similar occupational conditions. His views on the psychological and physical aspect of what would now be called work related upper limb disorders were very advanced for his time.

**Guillain-Barre Syndrome** – This is a polyneuropathy usually described as an acute infective polyneuritis. It is caused by inflammation of the spinal nerves soon after their formation at the junction of the nerve roots. All four limbs may be involved simultaneously. Sensory loss may involve the limbs or may spread to the trunk. If death from respiratory paralysis is prevented the outlook is good.

**Health and Safety at Work Act 1974** – The Health & Safety at Work Act (1974) requires employers to do all that is reasonably practicable to safeguard their employees health. Since the beginning of 1993 management of health and safety regulations further specify that the employer makes suitable and sufficient assessments of hazards and risk in the workplace and ensures that appropriate health surveillance is carried out. No doubt this will be expanded with regard to the European Community Directive on physical hazards in the workplace.

**Heuristic** – A branch of logic dealing with discovery and invention usually used, in the medical context, to find out answers.

**Hyperaemia** – An abnormal or excessive accumulation of blood.

**Hyperalgesia** – An abnormal or excessive sensation, or heightened sensitivity, of the nerves. Hypoalgesia is the opposite and both have been grouped to mean 'altered peripheral neural sensibility'

**Hyperaesthesia** – An increased pain response.

**Hypoaesthesia** – A reduction in the sensation of pain.

**Inappropriate Pain Syndrome** – This is a condition where the symptoms appear to be out of keeping with the physical findings and although the precipitating activity has stopped the pain persists. This pain is initially due to a physical cause – i.e. long periods of keyboard work – but later a secondary, psychological factor manifests itself. There are often good reasons for this. The persons concerned may have lost their jobs, incomes are reduced, they are unable to carry out many mundane, social and domestic activities, and the quality of their life changes for the worse. It is therefore, understandable that under these circumstances psychological problems develop and it is very easy to attribute the individual's problems to psychological causes and to forget the precipitating factor. The inappropriate pain syndrome undoubtedly has a psychological element to it which is difficult to reverse and is the reason why conventional treatment often fails and why pain clinics which practice cognitive therapy, which is a different approach to pain relief, can be successful.

**Iatrogenesis** – 'Iatrogenic' refers to the use of drugs and has come to mean that the drugs or treatments used have contributed not to the cure but to the continuing or worsening of the condition. In the 1980s Australian physicians coined the word 'iatrogenesis' believing that the principle cause of the 'epidemic' of 'RSI' in

Australia was due to poor diagnosis on the part off the physicians compounded by the wrong treatment, and the perpetuation of the idea of an epidemic supported by ongoing litigation.

**Intersection Syndromes** – This is also known as peritendinitis crepitus. It is often difficult to distinguish from de Quervain's tenovaginitis. It manifests itself as pain, crepitus and swelling in the forearm and tends to be work related in that it comes on when unaccustomed work is carried out, or following the return to work after a period of absence.

**Ischaemia** – Lacking in blood.

**'Kangaroo Paw'** – A derogatory term originating in Australia in the 1980s and refers to what was thought to be the over-diagnosis of 'RSI'.

**Keyboard Operator** – A person who uses a keyboard on a word processor or computer.

**Malingerophobia** – This is used to describe a situation in which doctors are so frightened of compensating malingerers that they are prepared to penalise the deserving majority.

**Marfan's Syndrome** – This is an inherited condition of collagen tissue which may have minimal or even advantageous affects on the individual or – at its extreme – can be a life threatening syndrome. As far as work related upper limb disorders are concerned lax joints (double joints) may be present in those of unusually tall build, possessed of an arm spread greater than their height, which can lead to joint and posture problems. Marfan's is probably the term given to an extensive family including many different types of collagen disorders.

**Morbidity** – The condition of being diseased. The morbidity rate is the percentage of people who are affected by a particular condition.

**Mortality** – The death rate for a particular condition.

**Motor Phenomena** – Loss of power in the hands and arms without any significant associated muscle wasting. It may also be associated with poor co-ordination, fatigue on repetitive movements, and loss of fine movements.

**MRI Scans** – Magnetic Resonance Imaging. A non invasive method of imaging the body and its organs. The body is placed in a magnetic field which causes certain atomic nuclei to align in the direction of the field. Pulses of radio frequency are then applied and interpretation of the frequencies absorbed and re-emitted allows an image of any body place to be built up.

**Musculo-Skeletal** – This refers to the skeleton and soft tissue of the body and is a non specific term, often used when taking a medical history or carrying out a physical examination, to describe the condition of the patient's bones, muscles, tendons and nerves.

**Myalgia** – An abnormal state of the muscles characterised by pain and cramp.

**Myelopathy** – A degenerative condition of the muscles.

**Myofascial Pain Syndrome (MPS)** – This describes a regional muscle pain disorder characterised by localised muscle tenderness and pain associated with a trigger point.

**Myofascial Trigger Points** – This is defined as a hyper irritable spot which is painful on compression and can give rise to referred pain, tenderness and autonomic phenomena.

**Negligence** – An employer can be sued for compensation for industrial disease or injury but, for an action of negligence to succeed, it has to be proved that the job actually caused the disease, it could have been prevented by the assessment and monitoring of working conditions and that a good employer would thus have prevented it.

**Neuralgia** – An acute pain in a nerve or a series of nerves especially in the head or face.

**Neurasthenia** – An old fashioned unspecific word usually meaning weakness of the nervous system or nervous exhaustion. Not a phrase that is used much these days.

**Neurolemma** – A membranous sheath encasing a nerve.

**Neuro Muscular Junction** – The specialised area where a motor nerve ends in close proximity to the muscle membrane and is able to initiate muscle contraction.

**Noeiceptors** – Nerve endings which detect and respond to painful or unpleasant stimuli.

**Neuritis** – Inflammation of a nerve. This may be localised to one point of the body – as in sciatica – or it may be more generally known as multiple neuritis or polyneuritis.

**Neurodynamic Testing** – See Brachial Plexus and Adverse Neural Tension.

**Neurology** – The scientific study of the anatomy, physiology and pathology of the nerves.

**Neuroma** – A tumour of a nerve.

**Neuropath** – An abnormality within the nervous system. A person suffering from a nervous disorder or having abnormal nervous sensibility

**Neuropathy** – Any disease of the nervous system.

**Neurophysiology** – The physiology of the nervous system.

**Neuroplasticity** – A phrase used in defining the relationship between soft tissues and injuries to the central nervous system and of the peripheral nerves.

**Neuropsychology** – Psychology based upon the study of the nervous system.

**No Fault System** – This is a compensation scheme such as has been set up in New Zealand and Sweden where an insurance company pays compensation following diagnosis of injury. It is not necessary to prove negligence. The schemes are said to be quick and cheap to administer but have the disadvantage of not adapting quickly to new industrial diseases or compensating where there is only a probability that the problem is work related.

**Nosology** – The branch of medical science dealing with the systematic classification of diseases usually described as the nomenclature of disease.

**Nosophobia** – A morbid fear of disease.

**Osler, Sir William FRS (1849–1919)** – Regius professor of Medicine at Oxford. Author of the Principles and Practice of Medicine. Described pain affecting telegraphy workers.

**Osteoarthritis (OA)** – These are changes in the joints due to wear and tear associated, later, with changes in the synovial membranes and synovial fluids. It is a very common condition and all people as they get older have an element of osteoarthritis in some of their joints. Excessive occupational wear and can lead to OA at a much younger age than is normal.

**Overuse Syndrome** – This is a non specific term and describes the effects on the musculo-skeletal tissue of over-use or misuse of a joint or a tissue. The term is often used synonymously with 'Repetitive Strain Injury' or 'Work Induced Upper Limb Disorders' and similar terms in different countries.

**Painful Arch Syndrome** – This is a clinical syndrome characterised by pain in the shoulder and upper arm during abduction of the arm, with freedom from pain at the extremes of the range of movements. With the arm dependent the pain is absent but during abduction of the arm pain begins at about 45 degrees and persists through the arch of movement to about 160 degrees when it lessens or disappears. It can be caused by a number of different lesions to the shoulder muscles or joint capsule.

**Peritendinitis** – This is a typical reaction to repetitive movements of the wrist or hand and is a type of frictional tenosynovitis. Those tendons most affected are those of the deep muscles at the back of the forearm especially the extensors of the thumb and the radial extensors of the wrist. The pain appears after a period of unusual use of the hand or wrist and there is often a mild inflammatory reaction with swelling above the tendon and its coverings. On examination there may be localised swelling in the line of the affected tendons and a fine crepitation is felt over the area of inflammation.

**Phelan's Test** – Moving the wrist off neutral causes paraesthesia (pins and needles) in the distribution of the median nerve as in carpal tunnel syndrome.

**Prescribed Industrial Disease** – This is a condition which has been prescribed by the Industrial Injuries Advisory Council. Work related upper limb disorders may be prescribed as industrial disease but where the Council considers it could be caused by activities outside the workplace – and is not necessarily related to specific occupations – the injury is not prescribed. For example 'tennis elbow' (epicondylitis of the humerus) and 'frozen shoulder' (rotator cuff syndrome) in the Council's opinion are not prescribed as they are common in the general population and there is insufficient evidence to link them with specific occupational groups. Similarly, carpal tunnel syndrome is not covered. Disablement benefit may be paid only if work induced tenosynovitis has previously been diagnosed or if carpal tunnel syndrome arises from the use of hand held vibrating tools.

**Poore G.V. Dr** – Physician at University College, London. Wrote about writer's cramp in 1877.

**Psycho-Social Phenomena** – An unspecific term often used where an upper limb problems is thought not to be organic but to be related to the psychological state of the individual.

**Ramazzini** – Bernardino Ramazzini (1633–1714) is described as the father of occupational medicine. He was professor of medicine at the University of Modena and later in Padua. His great work *De Morbis Artificum Diatriba* is one of the most important books in the history of medicine. He was well in advance of his times and investigated the medical aspects of a great many of the occupations then current in Italy. He stated:

> 'Medicine, like jurisprudence, should make a contribution to the well being of workers and see to it that, so far as possible, they should exercise their callings without harm.'

**Radicular Pain** – As far as the upper limbs are concerned this is pain due to pressure or entrapment of the cervical nerve roots. The nerve roots can be nipped by being stretched over a disc herniation or compressed by disc material or bony encroachment into the intervertebral foramen.

**Radiculopathy** – This refers to the actual pathological process which causes the radicular pain. It may be due to disease, compression, or reduction in local blood supply by other causes.

**Radial Tunnel Syndrome** – This is caused by pressure on the posterior interosseous nerve within the tunnel formed by five anatomical structures at the lateral epicondyle (outer aspect of the elbow) and is the explanation for one of the many causes of pain in the elbow. Diagnostically the pain is worsened if the middle finger is pressed backwards and improved by anaesthetic block within the radial tunnel. The syndrome may be work related and tends to improve with rest. Surgery may help by decompressing the posterior interosseous nerve within the radial tunnel. But it may not. The use of local anti-inflammatory drugs may also be beneficial.

**Raynaud's Phenomenon or Disease** – This was named after Dr Maurice Raynaud who in 1862 wrote a thesis entitled *De L' Asphyxia Locale et de la Gangrene Symetrique des Extremities*. It is peripheral vascular disturbance probably due to abnormal activity of the vasoconstrictor nerves which leads to constriction of the arteries in the fingers and thumb, precipitated by cold, emotion and by many other factors (see Vibration White Finger). The digits become blanched, painful and cold and in severe cases it can lead to gangrene. It also follows any hand surgery in about 2% to 3% of patients and there is no way of predicting who will be affected.

**Referred Pain** – This pain manifesting itself at a distance from the actual nerve root compression or nerve injury.

**Reflex Sympathetic Dystrophy** – This is an unpleasant complication which may follow fractures about the wrist. In its early stages the condition is characterized by swelling of the soft tissues, exquisite tenderness to pressure, and pain on motion. Later, circulatory changes occur in the soft tissues and bone, the skin becomes purplish and cold, and there may be excessive perspiration. Much later the joints of the fingers and wrists become increasingly stiff and even the shoulder and elbow may be affected secondarily from voluntary immobilization of the arm in one position. X-rays reveal a mottled decalcification or osteoporosis of the bones. No treatment is entirely satisfactory but minimal immobilization with active and passive exercises, sympathetic blocks, and occupational and physical therapy seem to be as effective as any other treatment. Until symptoms and signs are relatively static, or a definite improvement is apparent, surgery should be delayed.

**Regional Allodynia – Regional Pain Disorder** – Diffuse pain and tenderness outside any single anatomical structure or boundary, worse with hand use but with little improvement in pain free function, even after prolonged reduction in hand use activities, even in the absence of any definable rheumatological or orthopaedic. This is a condition of unknown causation.

**Regional Pain Syndrome** – Pain often referred from a central point where there is an element of nerve entrapment.

**Repetitive Strain Injury** – This is the term previously given to damage to muscles, nerves, tendons, tendon sheaths or other soft tissues resulting from overuse or misuse usually in the upper limbs. The lower limbs, back, shoulders and other parts of the body however, can also be affected. Unfortunately the term does not conform to conventional criteria for the description of disease and this can lead to confusion – particularly if litigation is contemplated – for it implies the existence of a physical condition with an identifiable cause.

Physical signs may be imprecise or absent, the word 'strain' is not used in its true mechanical sense – but in a lay sense – and 'injury' suggests a single culpable event.

However, the term 'RSI' has wide understanding in lay circles and the RSI Associations do valuable work for their members and it is reasonable that the term continues – if only to prevent it being replaced by something equally imprecise and providing the qualifications to its use are appreciated.

**Rheumatoid Arthritis (RA)** – Rheumatoid arthritis is a chronic non bacterial inflammation of joints which causes thickening of the synovial membrane and chronic inflammatory changes. The articular cartilages are later softened and eroded. Osteoarthritis may be due to occupational hazards leading to wear and tear in the joints but rheumatoid arthritis is a disease without any known occupational associations.

**Rotator Cuff Syndrome** – This refers to a cuff of soft tissue over the tip of the shoulder made up of the supra-spinatus tendon and the adjoining flat tendons which are blended together to form what is often called the rotator cuff. Injury to the cuff produces pain at the tip of the shoulder reflecting down the upper arm, and the inability to abduct the arm without pain.

**Sclerotome** – This describes the segmental localisation of symptoms in the upper and lower limbs. It is used to distinguish the pattern of referred pain from the dermatome of nerve root stimulation. Both sclerotomes and dermatomes have segmental characteristics but sclerotomes are more diffuse and are not associated with the specific sensory and motor disturbances of dermatomes. It may be associated with sweating, pallor and nausea.

**Sensory Phenomena** – This refers to sensory symptoms such as numbness and tingling. It is used in the evaluation and diagnosis of neurological disorders.

**Social Iatrogenesis** – A phrase used in Australia during the 1980s when there was a good deal of criticism of the diagnosis of 'RSI' and it was thought that the discussions in the press and the media generally led to a heightened awareness of the dangers of RSI which in itself led to more cases. It was described as 'propaganda in the pursuit of litigation.'

**Somatic Dysfunction** – Some form of disturbance of the central nervous system which is not demonstrable by contemporary scientific investigative techniques. It is thought to be one of the causes of muscle tenderness in referred pain in the upper limbs.

**Speed's Test** – A test for biceps tendinitis. Flexion of the elbow against resistance produces pain of the long head of the biceps tendon.

**Sudomotor** – Sweating.

**Sudeck's Atrophy** – See: Reflex Sympathetic Dystrophy

**Supraspinatus Tendinitis** – Pain at the tip of the shoulder due to inflammation of the supraspinatus muscle or degeneration of the tendon fibres. There is often minimal pain when the arm is dependent, but during abduction there is shoulder pain at about 45 degrees which persists through the arch of movement until about 160 degrees at which point the pain lessens or disappears.

**Syndrome** – A group of signs and symptoms which when present together allow the description and naming of a particular disease process.

**Synovial Membrane** – The lining of a joint tendon sheath, or bursae. When making a diagnosis of tenosynovitis care must be taken to ensure that this term is used only in the presence of synovium.

**Synovial Fluid** – The synovial membrane produces a viscid fluid called synovial fluid (synovia) which acts as a lubricant allowing the free movement of the tendon within its sheath or the structures within a joint. Synovial fluid may help to nourish the articular cartilages and is capable of absorbing micro-organisms and the cartilaginous debris which results from ordinary wear and tear.

**Telegraphist's Cramps** – This is another of the old names for a condition which would today probably be described as writer's cramp or a work related upper limb disorder.

**Tendinopathy** – This refers to pathological conditions in the hand, wrist and forearm which are frequently the result of overuse and as such are work related upper limb disorders. They include tenosynovitis, de Quervain's tenovaginitis and various pathological conditions of the extensor and flexor tendons including tennis and golfer's elbow and many others.

**Tendinitis** – Inflammation followed by thickening of the tendons producing symptoms of pain and local tenderness similar to those of tenosynovitis. The thickening and scarring may become so severe that the tendon may be unable to move freely within the synovial sheath and the effected fingers or limbs are prevented from going through their normal range of movements. Trigger finger is an example.

**Tenosynovitis** – Inflammation of the thin synovial lining of a tendon sheath. It may be caused by a mechanical irritation. Where there is excessive friction from overuse the synovial sheath is mildly inflamed and there is an exudate of watery fluid within it. If identified early on the condition can be cured but eventually the sheaths and the tendons become inflamed and scared and there may be permanent irreversible damage. The most affected tendons are the radial extensors and the abductors of the wrist and thumb.

In the list of prescribed diseases it is number A8.

**TENS** – This stands for Transcutaneous Electrical Nerve Stimulation which is created by a small mobile pack which can be strapped to the arm. These machines can be borrowed or hired from some Departments of Physiotherapy and have the advantage of being under the patient's own control. This is one of the few forms of treatment which seems to give real relief to work related upper limb disorder sufferers.

**Thoracic Outlet Syndrome** – This rare condition is caused by nerve compression in the root of the neck by anatomically abnormal structures.

**Tinel's Sign** – A compressed nerve has a lower threshold to mechanical stimulation so percussion over a site of entrapment elicits a 'Tinel's Sign'. Tapping over, or putting pressure on, the median nerve may provoke the sensory symptoms of carpal tunnel syndrome or a Tinel's sign. This is not a very reliable test.

**Trigger Finger and Thumb** – This is characterised by tenderness at the base of the affected finger and 'locking' of the finger in full extension. The locking can either be overcome by effort or by extending the finger passively with the other hand. When flexion is released there is a distinct snap and on examination there is a palpable nodule, usually slightly tender, at the base of the affected finger or thumb. There are changes over the mouth of the fibrous flexor sheath which are caused by the tendons becoming 'wasted' opposite the constriction and swollen proximal to it.

**Ultra Sound** – One of the non invasive means of investigations used in a department of clinical radiology. Also one of the treatments used by physiotherapists to give symptomatic relief of work related upper limb disorders.

**Unfair Dismissal** – Workers have to be employed by the same employer for two years – soon to be reduced to one year – before they have the right to take a case for unfair dismissal to the Industrial Tribunal.

**Vibration White Finger Syndrome** – This is a condition in which the control of the blood vessels to the fingers is disturbed and one or more of the fingers become white as the blood supply is closed off. The hands become clumsy particularly in cold weather or cold working conditions. It is progressive and irreversible and has been a prescribed disease since 1985.

**Visual Display Unit** – The screen which is part of the computer or word processor.

**Wartenberg's Syndrome** – This is also known as superficial radial neuropathy and is due to compression of the sensory branch of the radial nerve above the wrist. This can be as a result of a tight wrist watch strap, the use of hand cuffs, splints, operations around the wrist, or trauma to the wrist.

**Wigley Test** – This measures the ability of the patient to carry out fine movements. The time taken to touch all fingers with the thumb four times in rapid sequence in a limb thought to be suffering from an overuse syndrome and compared with the other (unaffected) limb.

**WRULD** – Work related upper limb disorders. This describes a range of conditions characterised by discomfort or persistent pain in muscles, tendons and other soft tissues with or without clearly visible injury or physical signs. It includes tenosynovitis, carpal tunnel syndrome, tennis and golfer's elbows, and vibration white finger. They may be caused or aggravated by rapid or repetitive movements, poor posture and possibly psycho-social factors. WRULD has been suggested as an alternative term to Repetitive Strain Injury which is now thought to be a misleading term. The symptoms and signs as described in WRULDs may be unrelated to work and accurate diagnose is essential if litigation is contemplated.

**Yergason's Test** – A test for biceps tendinitis. Resisted supination of the forearm with the elbow flexed at 90 degrees produces pain over the long head of the biceps tendon.

# References


1. Ohara H., Aroyama H. and Itani T.: Health hazard among cash register operators and the effects of improved working conditions. *J Hum Ergol (Tokyo)*, 1976, *5*, 31–40.
2. Hunting W., Grandjean E. and Maeda K.: Constrained postures in accounting machine operators. *Appl. Ergonomics*, 1980, *11*: 145–9
3. Nagira T., Suzuki J., Ol Y., *et al*.: Cervicobrachial and low back disorders among school lunch workers and nursery school teachers in comparison with cash register operators. *J Hum Ergol (Tokyo)*, 1981, *10*, 117–24.
4. Lapoajarvi T., Juorinka I., Virolainen M. and Holmberg M.: Prevalence of tenosynovitis and other injuries of the upper extremities in repetitive work. *Scand J Work Environ Health*, 1979, *5 (suppl 3)*, 48–55.
5. Maeda K.: Occupational cercvicobrachial disorder and its causative factors. *J Hum Ergol (Tokyo)*, 1977, *6*, 193–202.
6. Ohara H., Nakagiri S., Itani T., *et al*.: Occupational health hazards resulting from elevated work rate situations. *J Hum Ergol (Tokyo)*, 1976, *5*, 173–82.
7. Ohara H., Itani T. and Aoyama H.: Prevalence of occupational cervicobrachial disorder among different occupational groups in Japan. *J Hum Ergol (Tokyo)*, 1982, *11*, 55–63.
8. Nakaseko M., Tokunga R. and Hosokawa M.: History of occupational cervicobrachial disorder in Japan. *J Hum Ergol (Tokyo)*, 1982, *11*, 7–16.
9. Arndt R.: Working posture and musculoskeletal problems of visual display terminal operators: review and reappraisal. *Am Ind Hyg Assc J*, 1983, *44*, 437–46.
10. Harris J.E.: Repetition strain injury. Proceedings of the Royal Australian College of Surgeons/Royal Australian College of Physicians Seminar, *Disability in the Workforce*. Melbourne: RACS/RACP 1984.

11. Hadler N.M.: Industrial rheumatology. Three Australian and New Zealand experiences with arm pain and backache in the workplace. *Med J Aust*, 1986, *144*, 191–5.
12. National Occupational Health and Safety Commission: *Interim Report of the RSI Committee*. Canberra: Australian Govt Publishing Service, 1985.
13. Taylor R. and Pitcher M.: Medical and ergonomic aspects of an industrial dispute concerning occupational related conditions in data process operators. *Community Health Study*, 1984, *8*, 172–80.
14. *Hunters Diseases of Occupation,* 5th edition, 1969.
15. Holbrook T.L., Grazier K., Kelsey J. and Stauffer R.: *The frequency of Occurrence, Impact and Costs of Selected Musculoskeletal Conditions in the United States*. Chicago: American Academy of Orthopaedic Surgeons, 1984, 1–87.
16. Bureau of Labour Statistics: *Occupational Injuries and Illnesses in the United States by Industry 1989*. US Dept of Labour, Bulletin 2379. Washington, DC: US Government Printing Office, 1991.
17. Rempel D.M., Harrison R.J. and Barnhart, S.: Work related cumulative trauma disorders of the upper extremity *JAMA*, 1992, *267*, 838–842.
18. Mallory M. and Bradford H.: An invisible workplace hazard gets harder to ignore. *Business Week*, 30 January 1989, 92–93.
19. News Report. *Daily Telegraph,* July 1998
20. Association of Schools of Public Health/National Institute for Occupational Safety and Health: *Proposed National Strategies for the Prevention of Leading Work related Diseases and Injuries: Part 1*. Washington, DC: Association of Schools of Public Health, 1986, 19.
21. Health & Safety Commission: *Health & Safety Statistics, statistical supplement to the 1994–5 annual report*. Sudbury, Suffolk: HSE Books, 1995.

22. Greening J. and Lynn B.: Vibration sense in the upper limb in patients with repetitive strain injury and a group of at-risk office workers. *Int Arch Occup Environ Health*, 1997.
23. Thompson A.R., Plewes L.W. and Shaw E.G.: Peritendinitis crepitans and simple tenosynovitis: a clinical study of 544 cases in industry. *Br J Ind Med,* 1951, *8*, 150–9.
24. *Grays Anatomy,* 30th edition, 1949.
25. *Weekly Law Reports,* 10th July 1998. *Pickford* v. *Imperial Chemical Industries* (House of Lords).
26. Silverstein B.A., Fine L.J. and Armstrong T.J.: Occupational factors and carpal tunnel syndrome. *Am J Ind Med*, 1987, *11*, 343–358.
27. American Association of Electrodiagnostic studies in carpal tunnel syndrome: summary statement. *Muscle Nerve*, 1993, *16*, 1390–1391.
28. AAEM Quality Assurance Committee: Literature review of the usefulness of nerve conduction studies and electromyography for the evaluation of patients with carpal tunnel syndrome. *Muscle Nerve*, 1993, *16*, 1392–1414.
29. Armstrong T.J. and Silverstein B.A.: Upper extremity Pain in the Workplace – Role of Usage in Causality. In: N.M. Hadler (ed.), *Clinical Concepts in Regional Musculo–skeletal Illness*. Orlando: Grune & Stratton, 1987, 333–354.
30. Smith E.M., Sonstegard D.A. and Anderson W.H. Jr.: Carpal tunnel syndrome: contribution of flexor tendons. *Arch Phys Med Rehabil*, 1977, *58*, 379–385.
31. Gelberman R., Hergenroeder P., Hargens A. and Lundborg G., *et al.*: The carpal tunnel syndrome. A study of carpal tunnel pressures. *J Bone Joint Surg (Am)*, 1981, *61*, 380–383.
32. Ski M., Zeiss J., Ebraheim N.A. and Jackson W.T.: Carpal tunnel changes and median nerve compression during wrist flexion and extension seen by magnetic resonance

imaging. *J Hand Surg*, 1990, *15A*, 934–939.

33. Brain W.R., Wright A. and Wilkinson M.: Spontaneous compression of both median nerves in carpal tunnel. *Lancet*, 1947, *1*, 277–282.
34. Lundborg G., Gelberman R., Minteer-Convery M. and Lee V.F., *et al.*: Median nerve compression in the carpal tunnel: the functional response to experimentally induced controlled pressure. *J Hand Surg*, 1982, 7, 252–259.
35. Szabo R.M. and Chidgey L.K.: Stress carpal tunnel pressure in patients with carpal tunnel syndrome and normal patients. *J Hand Surgery*, 1989, *14A*, 624–627.
36. Faithfull D.K., Moir D.H. and Ireland J.: The micropathology of the typical carpal tunnel syndrome. *J Hand Surg*, 1986, *11B*, 131–132.
37. Feldman R.G., Travers P.H., Chinico-Post J. and Keyserling W.M.: Risk assessment in electronic workers: carpal tunnel syndrome. *J Hand Surg (Am)*, 1987, *12*, 849–55.
38. Birkbeck M.Q. and Beer T.C.: Occupation in relation to the carpal tunnel syndrome. *J Hand Surg (Br)*, 1988, *13*, 167–70.
39. Harrington J.M., Carter J.T., Birrell, L. and Gompertz D.: Surveillance case definitions for work related upper limb pain syndromes. *Occup Environ Med*, 1998, *55*, 264–271.
40. Harrington J.M., Gompertz D. and McCaig R.H.: Repetitive Strain Injuries. *Lancet*, 1997, *349*, 1701–2.
41. Hodgson J.T., Jones J.R., Elliot R.C., *et al.*: *Self Reported Work Related Illness*. Sudbury, Suffolk: HSE Books, 1993 (Research paper 33.).
42. Selvaratnam P.J., Glasgow E.F. and Matyas T.: Differential strain produced by the brachial plexus tension test on C5 to T1 nerve roots. In: Jones, H.M., Jones, M.A. and Milde, M.R. (eds.), *Proceedings of the sixth biennial conference of the Manipulative Therapists' Association of Australia*. Adelaide: 1989, 167–172.

43. Karlsson J. and Ollander B.: Muscle metabolites with exhaustive static exercise of different durations. *Acta Physiol. Scand*, 1972, *86*, 309–14.
44. Bjorksten A. and Ionsson B.: Endurance limit of force in long-term intermittent static contractions. *Scand J Work Environ Health*, 1977, *3*, 23–7.
45. Onishi N., Sakai K. and Kogi K.: Arm and shoulder muscle load in various keyboard operating jobs of women. *J Hum Ergol (Tokyo)*, 1982, *11*: 89–97.
46. Vollestad N.K. and Sejerstad O.M.: 1988 Biochemical correlates of fatigue. *Eur J Appl Physiol.*, *57*, 336–347.
47. Edwards R.H.T.: 1988 Hypotheses of peripheral and centra mechanisms underlying occupational muscle pain and injury. *Eur J Appl Physiol.*, *57*, 275–281.
48. Friden J.: Muscle soreness after exercise: implications of morphological changes. *Int J Sports Med*, *5*, 57–66.
49. Larsson S.E., Bengtsson A., Bodegard L., Henriksson K.G. and Larsson J.: Muscle changes in work related chronic myalgia. *Acta Orthop Scand*,1988, *59*, 552–556.
50. Quintner J. and Elvey R.: The Neurogenic Hypothesis of RSI Working Paper no. 24, *National Centre for Epidemiology and Population Health*. Australian National University May 1991.
51. Grandjean E.: Postural problems at office work stations. In: Grandjean E. (ed.), *Ergonomics and Health in Modern Offices*. London: Taylor and Francis, 1969, 444–5.
52. Bjelle A., Hagberg M., Michaelson G.: Clinical and ergonomic factors in prolonged shoulder pain among industrial workers. *Scand J Work Environ Health*, 1979, *5*, 205–10.
53. Armstrong T.J., Foulke J.A., Joseph B.S. and Goldstein S.A.: Investigation of cumulative trauma disorders in a poultry processing plant. *Am Ind Hyg Assoc J.*, 1982, *43*, 103–116.
54. Leao L.: de Quervain's stenosing tenovaginitis. A clinical

and anatomical study. *J Bone Joint Surg (Am)*, 1958, *40*, 1063–70.

# Useful Addresses

As has been explained elsewhere the term Repetitive Strain Injury or RSI is not now generally used by medical practitioners – Work Related Upper Limb Disorders, WRULDs, being the term of choice in the United Kingdom. However, RSI is a term well known and widely understood by the lawyers and the national and locally organised 'RSI' Associations which do such excellent work and it is wise to continue the use of this well known and well publicised RSI name: to change now would be of benefit to no one. I have therefore, continued with the use of the term RSI in this list of useful addresses as that is the name many organisations choose to use.

**RSI Association**
Chapel House,
152 – 156 High Street,
Yiewsley,
West Drayton,
Middlesex UB7 7BE.
Tel: 01895 431 134 (Mon to Fri 11.30 am to 4 pm, answer phone other times) for details of the information pack and membership costs. Newsletters are published quarterly, containing local support group contact numbers.

The RSI Association provides invaluable help and information. They offer an excellent information pack. Sending for it is a good first step for anyone newly afflicted. Add a little extra if you can – the RSI Association is in need of funds. If you also become a member, you receive a quarterly newsletter, and can attend the AGM at which invited speakers talk about aspects of RSI. The RSI Association have a list of local support groups which is included in the information pack. This is an organisation well worth supporting both morally and financially.

**Pain Management Clinic**
St. Thomas's Hospital,
Lambeth Palace Road,
London SE1 7EH.
Tel: 0171 928 9292.
Fax: 0171 922 8079
This clinic, which is run by Dr Charles Pither, specialises in management of chronic pain, and many of those referred to it are suffering from WRULDs. The approach is holistic, involving physiotherapy, ergonomics, exercise and pain management. There is a long waiting list but their results are good.

**The Pain Society**
9 Bedford Square,
London WClB 3RA.
For a List of pain clinics and a leaflet about how pain clinics treat chronic pain, write to the Pain Society enclosing a stamped address envelope.

**Chartered Society of Physiotherapists**
14 Bedford Row,
London WC4 4ED.
Tel: 0171 242 1941.
They can put patients in touch with a physiotherapist experienced in the treatment of WRULDs.

**Bradford Occupational Health Project and Bradford RSI Support Group**
Myrtle Road Surgery,
23 Harrogate Road,
Bradford,
BD2 3DY.
Tel: 01274 626 191.

**The British School of Osteopathy**
1–4 Suffolk Street,
London SW1.
Tel: 0171 930 9254.

**The Society of Teachers in Alexander Technique**
20 London House,
266 Fulham Road,
London SW10 9EL.
Tel: 0171 351 0828

**Interact**
Premier House,
313 Kilburn Lane,
London W9 3EG.
Tel: 0181 968 6633.

**Musicians & Keyboard Clinic**
7 Park Crescent,
London W1.
Tel: 0171 436 5961.

**Healthline** – A freephone health information service
Tel: 0800 66 55 44
You can ring during office hours to ask questions on any health subject. You can ask them to send you an information sheet. Within London, the service is partly automated. During office hours the line is answered in person. Outside those times, if you have a touch tone telephone you can listen to a pre-recorded tape on any of several dozen subjects, by inputting the tape number to the automated answering service. Tapes of interest to WRULD sufferers are: 353 Repetitive Strain Injury, 319 Carpal Tunnel Syndrome, 174 Pain Clinics

**National Bureau for Students with Disabilities**
336 Brixton Road,
London SW9 7AA.
Tel: 0171 274 0565.

**SKILL**
SKILL advise disabled students on how to get help to enable them to continue with their studies. They produce a set of Information Sheets, one of which is on 'Specialist Equipment in Education: sources of help and information' This gives very clear details of the Disabled Student Allowances and how to apply.

**NUJ RSI Sufferers Group**
National Union of Journalists,
Acorn House,
314–320 Gray's Inn Road,
London WClX 8DP.
Tel: 01424 225 610.

**City Centre**
32–35 Featherstone Street,
London ECIY 8QX.
Tel: 0171 608 1338.
City Centre are funded by the London Borough Grants Committee. They provide advice on office health and safety, and publish a number of newsletters and booklets including *An Office Worker's Guide to Repetitive Strain Injury*.

**London Hazards Centre**
Interchange Studios Dalby Street,
London NW5 3NQ.
Tel: 0171 267 3387.
They provide advice and information on all aspects of health and safety at work, including RSI risks. The Centre has an

extensive library and publishes a very informative booklet on RSI.

**Camden & Islington Occupational Health Project**
St. Pancras Hospital,
4 St. Pancras Way,
London NWl OPE.
Tel: 0171 383 0997.
Advice, information and a newsletter and an extensive RSI library is available to those who live or work in the London Borough of Camden or Islington.

**Sheffield Occupational Health Project**
Mudford's Building,
37 Exchange Street,
Sheffield S2 5TR.
Tel: 01132 755 760.
Advice and information for people living in Sheffield. They produce some excellent leaflets and broadsheets with information on assessing jobs and works stations. Please send a large SAE.

**Manchester Area RSI Support and Action Group**
C/o Greater Manchester Hazard Centre,
23 New Mount Street,
Manchester M4 4DE.
Tel: 0161 834 5929.
A group for RSI sufferers in the Manchester area. Telephone helpline: Tuesdays 11.00 am to 2.00 pm.

**Health & Safety Executive**
Rose Court,
2 Southwark Bridge,
London SE1 9HS.
Tel: 0171 717 6000.

The Health & Safety Executive are the statutory body responsible for ensuring safety at the workplace, and hence the body responsible for ensuring that employers comply with the 'Display Screen Equipment Regulations (1992)'.

The HSE give general advice about the legal requirements. They also publish guides to preventing RSI, workstation set up, etc., and offer advice to employers. They have a very large library which is open to the public.

There are local HSE offices throughout the country, which are listed in the telephone directory.

Employment Medical Advisory Service

The Employments Medical Advisory Service is part of the HSE. They advise employees, employers, and doctors on the effects of particular kinds of work on the health. To contact EMAS ring your local HSE office. They will give the numbers of the EMAS office covering the area where you work.

**ACAS**
Clifton House,
83 Euston Road London,
NW1 2RB.
Tel: 0171 396 5100.

ACAS can tell about employment rights, if a worker is threatened with dismissal. They do not advise on individual cases over the telephone, but they can explain the law, and state in what circumstances it might be possible to bring a successful case of unfair dismissal. There are regional offices throughout the country listed in the telephone directory.

ACAS publish a number of reading lists, including one on Repetitive Strain Injury. Write to:

**ACAS Reader Ltd**
P.O. Box 404,
Leicester, LE4 9ZZ.
Tel: 01533 463346

Also available from ACAS, or actually published by the

Employment Department are two useful booklets: *Fair and Unfair Dismissal* and *Unfairly Dismissed?*. These booklets explain what is meant by 'unfair dismissal' – essential information for those who lose their jobs as a result of RSI.

**Trade Unions**

Unions can give advice on RSI and help deal with any problems at work. Many unions have produced their own reports and booklets on RSI. The TUC has recently conducted a campaign on RSI, 'Don't Suffer in Silence,' producing training materials for shop stewards and a seven point 'Call For Action' on Medical Responses to RSI. For further information contact:

**Trades Union Congress**
Congress House,
Great Russell Street,
London WClB 3LS.
Tel: 0171 636 4040.

**Association of Personal Injury Lawyers**
l0a Byard Lane,
Nottingham NG1 2GH.
Tel: 0115 958 0585.

**Allied Lawyers Response Team (ALeRT)**

ALeRT is a network of solicitors' firms around the country working as a team sharing evidence, tactics and skills through a central office. Member firms can offer free initial advice on RSI cases.

**The Accident Line (Freephone: 0500 192939)**

The Accident Line is a freephone number provided by the Law Society. Its purpose is to put members of the public who have suffered accident or personal injury in touch with a solicitor in their area who can offer free initial advice as to whether or not there is a viable case for compensation.

**Institute of Consumer Ergonomics**
University of Technology
Loughborough,
Leicestershire LEl1 3TU.
Tel: 01509 283300

**Institute of Occupational Medicine**
**Ergonomics Branch**
8 Roxborough Place,
Edinburgh EH8 9SU.
Tel: 0131 6675131

**Ergonomics Research Unit Robens Institute**
University of Surrey Guildford,
Surrey GU2 5XH.
Tel: 01483 300 800.
The Unit carries out research, runs training courses and conferences and has an ergonomics consultancy service.

**Institute of Occupational Ergonomics**
University of Nottingham,
University Park,
Nottingham NG7 2RD.

**The Ergonomics Society**
Loughborough University,
Loughborough.
Tel: 01509 611 088.

**Foundation for Communications for the Disabled**
25 High Street,
Woking Surrey GU21 1BW.
Tel: 01483 727848.

This organisation provides assessments and sells equipment.

**National Federation of ACCESS Centres**
Hereward College,
Bramston Crescent,
Tile Hill Lane,
Coventry CV4 9SW.
Tel: 01203 461 231
Individual assessments and advice on the use of enabling technology. There are centres located in various places throughout the country. The National Federation of Access Centres can tell which one is most suited to an individuals needs. Students who have been awarded the Disabled Students' Allowance can have the cost of an assessment refunded from the Allowance.
PACT and the Access to Work Scheme

The Access to Work Scheme was set up to provide help to anyone at a disadvantage in getting or keeping a job. Most significantly for RSI sufferers, this could include providing specialist computer equipment, e.g. a computer and software to enable an employee to use voice-input instead of a keyboard. Many RSI sufferers have been helped by this scheme.

Unfortunately, the rules were changed in December 1995 making it more difficult to qualify. Again in March 1996 there was another change. Anyone who is thinking of applying is advised to contact their local Disability Employment Advisor (in the nearest Job Centre) to find out the current rules.

**British Telecom**
Those who need to talk on the telephone without holding the receiver, DO NOT cradle the telephone handset between the neck and the shoulder – this is very bad for anyone, but especially if you suffer from RSI. If you rent the Converse 300 telephone from British Telecom they will give you a headset free of charge.
Tel: BT's freephone number 0800 800 150

# INDEX

# Notes

# Notes

# Notes

# Notes

# Notes

# Notes